D1029337

Tibetan Medicine and You

Tibetan Medicine and You

A Path to Wellbeing, Better Health, and Joy

Miriam E. Cameron
and Tenzin Namdul

*With a blessing by His Holiness
the 14th Dalai Lama*

ROWMAN & LITTLEFIELD
Lanham • Boulder • New York • London

Published by Rowman & Littlefield
An imprint of The Rowman & Littlefield Publishing Group, Inc.
4501 Forbes Boulevard, Suite 200, Lanham, Maryland 20706
www.rowman.com

6 Tinworth Street, London SE11 5AL, United Kingdom

British Library Cataloguing in Publication Information Available

Library of Congress Cataloging-in-Publication Data

978-1-5381-3501-3 (cloth)
978-1-5381-3502-0 (electronic)

∞™ The paper used in this publication meets the minimum requirements of
American National Standard for Information Sciences—Permanence of Paper for
Printed Library Materials, ANSI/NISO Z39.48-1992.

Contents

His Holiness the 14th Dalai Lama Message

Tibetan medicine is one of the greatest legacies of Tibetan Buddhist civilization. It is a system that can contribute substantially to maintaining a healthy mind and a healthy body. Like the traditional Indian and Chinese systems, Tibetan medicine views health as a question of balance. A variety of circumstances such as diet, lifestyle, seasonal, and mental conditions can disturb this natural balance, which gives rise to different kinds of disorders.

As an integrated system of health care, Tibetan medicine has served the Tibetan people well for many centuries, and I believe it still can provide much benefit to humanity at large. The difficulty we face in bringing this about is one of communication, for, like other scientific systems, Tibetan medicine must be understood in its own terms, as well as in the context of objective investigation.

Therefore, I welcome the establishment of the Tibetan Healing Initiative under the auspices of the Center for Spirituality & Healing, University of Minnesota. Working in collaboration with the Men-Tsee-Kang, the Tibetan Medical and Astro Institute here in Dharamsala, this represents a tremendously valuable opportunity to advance the study, research, and practice of Tibetan medicine involving physicians and scholars who have undergone traditional training as well as being exposed to a modern scientific environment. I am confident that this initiative will be of great benefit to serious students of Tibetan medicine and look forward to learning about the practical results of this admirable collaborative effort.

The Dalai Lama[1]

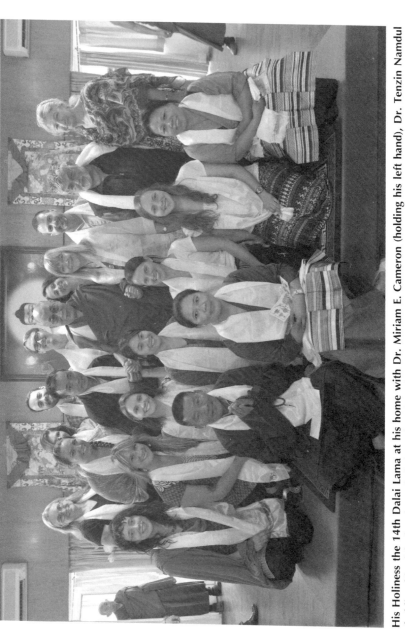

His Holiness the 14th Dalai Lama at his home with Dr. Miriam E. Cameron (holding his left hand), Dr. Tenzin Namdul (holding his right hand), and their University of Minnesota students, and staff in Dharamsala, India. *Source:* Official Photographer of His Holiness the Dalai Lama

Notes

Converting Tibetan Script to Roman Script

*W*e wrote Romanized Tibetan medical terms in italics. Tibetan medicine teaches that all phenomena are composed of five sources of energy, called elements. To name them, ancient Tibetans used terms from the natural world: **earth**, **water**, **fire**, **air**, and **space**. These five elements interact to form three principal energies: ***loong***, ***tripa***, and ***baekan***. To highlight their importance, we bolded each of the eight terms.

Many words from Tibetan Buddhism have become part of the English language. Examples are nirvana, karma, and bardo (Sanskrit: *nirvana*, *karma*, and Tibetan: *bar do*). We wrote these words without diacritics or italicization.

For readers' convenience, we converted Tibetan script to Roman script by spelling Tibetan terms the way they are pronounced. We intentionally used the simplified phonetic system adopted by the Men-Tsee-Khang (MTK) Translation Department in Dharamsala, India, in their translation of the *Gyueshi*,[1,2] the fundamental text of Tibetan medicine.[3]

The MTK's simplified phonetic system and the phonetic system developed by David Germano and Nicolas Tournadre[4] are based on the most commonly spoken dialect in Central Tibet and the exile Tibetan community. We chose the MTK's system, not the system by Germano and Tournadre, in order to maintain uniformity between the book, the MTK's English translation of the *Gyueshi*, and our other work in collaboration with the MTK.

Turrell Wylie[5] transliterated Tibetan script into Roman script that has less focus on pronunciation. We selected the MTK's system because it sounds closer to the spoken Central Tibetan Dialect than Wylie's transliteration does. Non-Tibetans outside of Tibet are most familiar with this dialect, and we don't want to confuse them.

The three columns in table 1 illustrate these different systems of converting Tibetan script to Roman script. For academics and researchers, we included Tibetan script, the phonetic system by Germano and Tournadre, and Wylie's transliteration, even though we didn't use them in the book.

Table 1. Tibetan Script, Men-Tsee-Khang Simplified Phonetic System Used in the Book, Phonetic System by Germano and Tournadre, and Wylie's Transliteration.

Tibetan Medical Terms in Tibetan Script	Simplified Phonetic System by MTK Translation Department (Bolded Text) and Phonetic System by Germano and Tournadre	Wylie's Transliteration
རླུང་	Loong / Lung	rLung
མཁྲིས་པ།	Tri pa	mKhrispa
བད་ཀན།	Baekan / be ken	Bad kan
ཉེས་པ་གསུམ།	Nyepa sum / nye' pa sum	Nye pa gsum
འབྱུང་བ་ལྔ།	Joong-wa-nya / Jungwa nga	Byung ba lnga
གསོ་བ་རིག་པ་	Sowa rik pa	Gso ba rig pa
རྒྱུད་བཞི།	Gyueshi / Gyü zhi	rgyud bzhi
སྲོག་འཛིན།	Sok zin / Sok dzin	Srog dzin
གྱེན་རྒྱུ	Gyen gyu	Gyen rgyu
ཁྱབ་བྱེད།	Kyab chay / Khyap je	Khyab byed
མེ་མཉམ།	May nyam / Me nyam	Me mnyam
ཐུར་སེལ།	Thoor sel / Tur sel	Thur sel
འཇུ་བྱེད།	Jhu chay / Ju je	Ju byed
མདངས་སྒྱུར།	Daang gyur / Dang gyur	Mdangs sgyur
སྒྲུབ་བྱེད།	Chup chay / Drup je	Sgrub byed
མཐོང་བྱེད།	Thong chay / Tong je	Mthong byed
མདོག་གསལ།	Dhok sel / Dok sel	Mdog gsal
རྟེན་བྱེད།	Then chay / Ten je	Rten byed
མྱག་བྱེད།	Nyak chey / Nyak je	Myag byed
མྱོང་བྱེད།	Nyong chay / Nyong je	Myong byed
ཚིམ་བྱེད།	Tseem chay / Tsim je	Tshim byed
འབྱོར་བྱེད།	Jor chay / Jor je	Byor byed
མ་རིག་པ།	Ma rig pa / Ma rik pa	Ma rig pa
ནང་ཆོས།	Nang choe / Nang cho	Nang chos
འཆི་བའི་འོད་སེལ།	Chi-way-voe-cel / chiwé ö sel	chi ba'i 'od sel
ཐུགས་དམ།	Tuk dam	Thugs dam
བར་དོ་ཐོས་གྲོལ་ཆེན་མོ།	Bar do tö dröl chen mo	Bar do thos grol chen mo
སྤྱི་གཙུག།	Chee tsuk / Chi tsuk	Spyi gtsug

Introduction

Tibetan Medicine: Self-Care and Integrative Care

Miriam E. Cameron

*A*ll of us want to be happy and avoid suffering. So why are many of us anxious, angry, depressed, and unfocused? We suffer from pain, insomnia, inflammations, hypertension, indigestion, and addictions. Our hearts are broken because life isn't going the way we want. The world seems to be getting worse, not better. Confused, we don't know who we are, why we are here, and how to live and die well. Tibetan medicine—Tibet's ancient, yet timely, science of healing—offers effective tools for transforming our suffering into healing and happiness.

Tibetan medicine teaches that the purpose of life is to be happy, and that after our basic needs are met, happiness results primarily from our own thinking. When challenges arise, we choose how to interpret them. We can wallow in negativity and get sick—or even sicker—in mind and body. Or we can decide to create health and happiness. Making good choices won't solve all of our problems but will produce better results than poor decisions do. At least, we won't make things worse.

Lotus seeds need mud to sprout, rise, and bloom. Tibetan medicine explains how to transform life's "mud" into nourishment that empowers us to flourish. It's up to us.

In this introduction, Dr. Tenzin Namdul and I will describe our perspectives on Tibetan medicine and why we wrote the book. First, I will explain why Tibetan medicine is effective for self-care and integrative care. A registered nurse, I have a PhD in nursing and philosophy/bioethics, as well as decades of experience in conventional health care, often called modern medicine, and Tibetan medicine. Nursing and Tibetan medicine are an excellent fit because they both focus on well-being and holistic healing.

Second, Tenzin will address the practice and relevance of Tibetan medicine. He is an experienced doctor of Tibetan medicine, called a *Menpa* in Tibetan and a Tibetan medicine practitioner in the United States. Recently, he completed his PhD in medical anthropology at Emory University in Atlanta.

Ideally, this book will advance interdisciplinary communication by serving as a bridge between conventional care and Tibetan medicine. Both traditions complement each other. They have the common goal of promoting healing and happiness.

WHAT IS TIBETAN MEDICINE?

Tibetan medicine is as old as Tibetan civilization. Over the millennia, Tibetan medicine has evolved into a profound science, art, philosophy, and psychology. A science, Tibetan medicine systematically investigates and explains the complex relationship between mind, body, and environment. An art, Tibetan medicine uses intuition and creativity. Tibetan medicine's philosophy and psychology are based on Tibetan Buddhism, a school of Buddhism that originated in India and later developed in Tibet. Tibetan medicine is universally applicable.

Tibetan medicine provides a cost-effective, holistic model for making informed decisions to create health and happiness. Health organizations are burdened by the cost of caring for those of us whose health problems result, in part, from our poor choices. Looking beyond conventional care provides answers to better health. Recent research publications, reviewed in chapter 15, are exploding with studies about the benefits of popular, inexpensive practices integral to Tibetan medicine. Using Tibetan medicine for self-care and integrative care promotes personal empowerment and offers more healing options than either tradition alone.

Self-care means to take action to preserve and improve health and happiness. Tibetan medicine teaches that each of us is born with a unique combination of energies called our constitution. To be healthy and happy, we must make informed decisions that support our constitution. Learning about our constitution will help us to choose the thoughts, food, behavior, environments, and other factors that keep our energies in balance.

Integrative care is an individual, coordinated, holistic, evidence-based health plan incorporating more than one healing system. As faculty at the University of Minnesota's Earl E. Bakken Center for Spirituality & Healing, Tenzin and I teach integrative care that includes conventional care and Tibetan medicine. Conventional care is better when emergency medicine, pharmaceuticals, technology, and surgery are needed. Tibetan medicine is most helpful to heal mind and body and to live and die well. The two traditions complement each other.

TIBETAN MEDICINE INTEGRATES ETHICS, SPIRITUALITY, AND HEALING

In 1994, I began studying Tibetan medicine after visiting South Korea and China. I was a postdoctoral fellow in nursing and cross-cultural ethics at the University of Minnesota, funded by the National Institute of Nursing Research at the National Institutes of Health. For years in my personal life, I had integrated conventional care with yoga and Ayurveda, healing traditions from India. Seoul National University College of Nursing invited me to give nine lectures about nursing ethics. To prepare, I read about Korean medicine. I came to see that my academic perspective based on conventional care was insufficient. To be holistic and comprehensive, I needed to integrate into my academic work the wisdom of traditional healing systems.

After leaving South Korea, I toured China and experienced Chinese medicine. Karma, our Tibetan tour guide, told me about Tibetan medicine, which is based on Tibetan Buddhism. Fascinated, I went to Tibet with Karma and other Americans in 1997. In Lhasa, I visited the Men-Tsee-Khang, the Tibetan Medical & Astrological Institute, where senior doctors explained the basic concepts of Tibetan medicine and did a consultation for me.

Back in Minnesota, I continued conducting ethics research studies as part of my postdoctoral work. I discovered that the findings were consistent with core teachings of Tibetan medicine. The diverse research participants were Americans with AIDS,[1] American elders and their families,[2] American nursing students,[3] and South Korean nursing students.[4] All of them addressed what Tibetan medicine calls karma, "As you sow, so shall you reap." They wanted to make choices that resulted in good consequences, not poor ones. For them, ethical, spiritual behavior promoted healing and happiness.

I realized that the findings from these four ethics studies and Tibetan medicine's core teachings support Virtue Ethics, a well-known ethical theory that I studied in graduate school. Plato and Aristotle, ancient Greek philosophers, taught that ethical behavior is essential for happiness or *eudaimonia*, a Greek word that means human flourishing. Aristotle wrote that Virtue Ethics consists of moral virtue and intellectual virtue. Moral virtue means to behave according to society's justifiable moral values (mores). Intellectual virtue has two components: (1) practical reasoning, or logic, that results in good choices and (2) contemplative reasoning, or meditation, that creates a vision for living according to the best ethical values. Without moral virtue and contemplative reasoning, practical reasoning may be blind and produce suffering, not happiness. Both moral virtue and intellectual virtue are prerequisites for happiness.

While agonizing over their ethical conflicts, the participants asked a question raised by Plato and Aristotle: "Why do we do what we say is wrong?" For example, some participants in the AIDS study told me in confidence that they engaged in unsafe sex and used intravenous drugs although they viewed these behaviors to be unhealthy and wrong. Plato and Aristotle used the term *akrasia* for a mind state in which we act against our own best judgment. We don't do what we say is right because we don't *really* know in our heart that the action is wrong.

Tibetan medicine sheds light on *akrasia*. We want to be happy and avoid suffering, but too often we are misguided. Out of ignorance, we mistakenly engage in negative thinking and make poor choices that produce suffering, not health and happiness. Even in challenging situations, we need to create meaning, seeing life as part of a bigger, purposeful picture. No matter what, we can choose to behave ethically, heal in mind if not in body, and be happy.

Likewise, yoga, India's precious gift to the world, teaches that ethics is crucial for healing and happiness. Patanjali, a sage in India two thousand years ago, wrote the *Yoga Sutra*, the basic text of yoga. Patanjali described Eight Limbs of Yoga, the first of which is ethics. By practicing the Limbs simultaneously, we create unity within and with everything. Ethics is the foundation for evolving spiritually and experiencing joy.

From a Native American perspective, health and happiness result from behaving with integrity. Our head, mouth, and heart are in alignment with each other and our best values. Suffering and dis-ease (lack of ease) develop if we don't think and say what our heart feels. Health and happiness are compromised when we know what our heart doesn't acknowledge.[5]

Judaism, Christianity, and Islam explain the relationship between ethics, spirituality, and healing. In the Bible, Moses instructed the Israelites to choose life, not death. As the Hebrew prophet Micah put it, we are required to behave with justice, mercy, and humility. Happiness results from ethical behavior that promotes healing of self, the community, and the world. The quintessential Jewish affirmation is *"L'chaim*: To life!" As a greeting, Jews, Christians, and Moslems say "Shalom," "Peace," and "Salam," which mean peace, health, and wholeness.

According to these traditions and the four ethics research studies, ethics, spirituality, and healing are not unrelated disciplines. Instead, they overlap. One without the others is insufficient. Behaving ethically—and helping to create an ethical society—is essential for health and happiness.

NEEDED: AN ACCESSIBLE BOOK IN ENGLISH ABOUT TIBETAN MEDICINE

In 2001, I published an integrative perspective in my book, *Karma and Happiness: A Tibetan Odyssey in Ethics, Spirituality, and Healing.*[6] His Holiness the 14th Dalai Lama wrote the foreword. I accepted a graduate faculty position at the Bakken Center and made my first of ten trips to the Men-Tsee-Khang, the Tibetan Medical & Astro-science Institute in Dharamsala, India, in the foothills of the spectacular Himalayas. Tenzin, a Men-Tsee-Khang faculty member, became my email contact person. Since then, Tenzin and I have collaborated on Tibetan medicine projects.

The Bakken Center partnered with the Dharamsala Men-Tsee-Khang and the Tibetan American Foundation of Minnesota to conduct two international Tibetan medicine conferences at the University of Minnesota. We held them in connection with teachings by the Dalai

Lama. The first conference generated such interest that I proposed teaching Tibetan medicine.

In 2002, Tashi Lhamo, *Menpa* from the Dharamsala Men-Tsee-Khang, immigrated to Minnesota, home of the second largest Tibetan community in the United States. Tashi, along with Tenzin in Dharamsala, helped me to create and teach two graduate courses:

1. "Traditional Tibetan Medicine: Ethics, Spirituality, & Healing." Since 2003, at least one thousand students have taken the course, now taught online.
2. "Tibetan Medicine, Ayurveda, & Yoga in India." Since 2005, about two hundred students have taken the course. The prerequisite is the Tibetan medicine course. Students travel to the Dharamsala Men-Tsee-Khang, where faculty members teach them a "Six-Day Intensive Course about Tibetan Medicine." They meet the Dalai Lama and/or other Tibetan scholars.

Nurses, physicians, and students in the health professions, diverse majors, and continuing education take these courses. The purpose isn't to become a Tibetan medicine practitioner. Qualified Tibetan medicine colleges require at least five years of study plus an internship with senior faculty. Instead, the courses teach students how to use Tibetan medicine for self-care and integrative care. In course reviews, students write that they learn to reduce stress, develop a positive focus, heal in mind and body, and be happy.

Colleagues and I organized our work involving Tibetan medicine into the Tibetan Healing Initiative (THI) at the Bakken Center. The Dalai Lama wrote blessings for THI and the Bakken Center. The two courses about Tibetan medicine led to two complementary graduate courses about Yoga, one of which is in India. Students study at Sadhaka Grama Ashram near Rishikesh and the Himalayan Institute Hospital Trust and Ayurveda Center in Jolly Grant. THI became part of the Yoga and Tibetan Medicine Focus Area, which I lead.

In 2005, I took seventeen University of Minnesota students to India. For the first time, we met Tenzin in person in New Delhi. He was charming, articulate, and informed. The following year, I invited him to be part of my second India group consisting of eighteen students. Since then, Tenzin has helped with each annual trip to Dharamsala, even after he immigrated to the United States to do undergraduate work at the University of Minnesota and graduate work at Emory University.

Finding textbooks for the Tibetan medicine graduate courses has been challenging. Most books about Tibetan medicine are written in Tibetan. Books written in English are too challenging for the students to understand and apply, don't meet academic standards, and/or are written by Tibetan medicine practitioners about how to practice Tibetan medicine professionally.

Tenzin and I decided to write a book for our students, health professionals, the general public, and everyone else interested in the healing power of Tibetan medicine. In India in 2006, Tenzin and I met to create a beginning table of contents. This book results from that meeting.

PURPOSE OF THE BOOK

The purpose of this book is to explain Tibetan medicine in easy-to-understand English while remaining authentic to the traditional teachings. Chapter 1 explains how to be happy. Everyone wants to be happy and avoid suffering. Each chapter builds on the previous chapters and becomes more profound. By continuing through the book, the reader develops a deeper understanding of Tibetan medicine.

Tibetan medicine is a huge discipline with many dimensions. This book does not address how to be a Tibetan medicine practitioner and to practice Tibetan medicine professionally. The book does not substitute for Tibetan medical colleges, Tibetan medicine practitioners, or other health professionals. Rather, this book explains in accessible English how to use Tibetan medicine for self-care and integrative care.

We wrote the book from three perspectives: (1) chapters 1 through 9 explain how readers can use Tibetan medicine for self-care; (2) chapters 10 through 14 describe the practice of Tibetan medicine to help readers include Tibetan medicine in their integrative care plans; and (3) chapter 15 addresses how health professionals, such as nurses and physicians, can integrate Tibetan medicine into their personal life and their evidence-based conventional care.

Although our work is scholarly, Tenzin and I avoided academic language in the book. We wrote in the second person to help you, the reader, understand and apply Tibetan medicine. Because text citations can be cumbersome to read, we primarily included them in chapter 15, where we reviewed the latest relevant research.

The book is based on the *Gyueshi*, the fundamental text of Tibetan medicine.[7,8,9] We consulted commentaries, Tibetan scholars, and Tibetan medicine faculty. Moreover, we included what we have learned about teaching Tibetan medicine to English-speaking students. To ensure scientific adequacy (the book accurately explains Tibetan medicine according to the *Gyueshi*), we used the rigorous phenomenological method that I created for my PhD dissertation research.[10] Colleagues and I have used this method successfully in many studies, including research involving Tibetan medicine.[11]

Meditation is essential to Tibetan medicine. In Tibetan tradition, the overall purpose of meditation is to tame the monkey mind and help it become a tool to create health and happiness. We included a meditation at the end of each chapter.

Our decades of experience with Tibetan medicine affirm for us the effectiveness of this ancient, timely tradition. Tibetan medicine explains how to create meaning and behave with integrity amid life's challenges. Cultivating compassion and wisdom transforms suffering into well-being, better health, and joy.

THANKS!

Thanks to Tenzin for years of collaborating with me on this book and other projects involving Tibetan medicine. Tenzin is an excellent Tibetan medicine practitioner, researcher, teacher, collaborator, and friend.

We couldn't write this book without generous assistance from many individuals and organizations. In particular, thanks to:

- Venerable Tibetan medicine practitioners (*Menpa*) for developing and preserving Tibetan medicine.
- Michael Ormond, my husband and soulmate, for participating with me in more than twenty-five years of Tibetan medicine adventures and for editing the book manuscript.
- University of Minnesota students for taking our courses.

- Tashi Lhamo, *Menpa*, BSN, RN, and Dechen Jamling, *Menpa*, BSN, RN, for doing Tibetan medicine consultations for our students.
- Tibetan organizations for collaborating with us: the Men-Tsee-Khang Medical College, Dharamsala, India; the Tibetan Medical College, Tso-Ngon (Qinghai) University, Amdo, Tibetan Plateau; the Men-Tsee-Kang, Lhasa, Tibet; the Tibetan American Foundation of Minnesota; and the Kunde Institute, Daly City, California.
- Mary Jo Kreitzer, director of the Bakken Center, and other colleagues who work closely with us: Kit Breshears, Pamela Cherry, Erin Fider, Dianne Lev, Susan O'Connor-Von, Christina Owen, Katie Schuver; Penny and Bill George, philanthropists, for sending donations with our India groups to the Men-Tsee-Khang, Tibetan Delek Hospital, and Tibetan Children's Villages in Dharamsala; Mariah Snyder, professor (retired), University of Minnesota School of Nursing (my alma mater), and other nursing faculty for teaching me how to practice integrative nursing.
- Swami Veda Bharati, my late yoga guru, and my teachers of Tibetan Buddhism and Judaism for explaining that God is all the conscious energy in the universe, not an anthropomorphic being. As manifestations of this energy, all of us are responsible to heal ourselves and the world.

A special thanks to the Dalai Lama for writing,

Tibetan medicine is far more advanced in the understanding of the nature of mind than Western medicine. . . . Without mixing the two approaches, and without saying one is better than the other, both schools should work together in order to find ways of understanding each other and thus boost the effectiveness of the two healing techniques.[12]

In this spirit, Tenzin and I wrote the book to benefit all beings.

The Practice and Relevance of Tibetan Medicine

Tenzin Namdul

This book largely came about because of Dr. Miriam Cameron's undying passion and perseverance. I first met Mim (what most people call her) and her husband, Michael Ormond (Mike), in person in New Delhi, India, on a cold evening in late December 2005. Mim and Mike were with a group of students from the University of Minnesota. I went to see them as a representative of the Men-Tsee-Khang, the Tibetan Medical & Astrological Institute in Dharamsala, India. We hit it off right away. For the next three weeks, I accompanied the group in their quest to learn more about Tibetan medicine, Ayurveda, and yoga. We were interested in finding out how these traditional healing systems speak to each other and to modern health-care systems.

Because of an accident, I first was exposed to the benefits of Tibetan medicine. While growing up in India, I wanted to study Western medicine. However, this endeavor was not feasible because of the unimaginable cost of medical school and the severe lack of scholarship funds for Tibetan refugees at that time. A good friend told me about the Dharamsala Men-Tsee-Khang. He said that applicants must pass the entrance exam and be admitted to the medical college. Then they receive funding for the six-year program to become a doctor of Tibetan medicine.

The Men-Tsee-Khang Medical College accepted me and gave me funding. As a medical student, I wasn't sure why I was there until I had a serious accident during an herbs-collection field trip near Rohtang Pass in the Himalayas. This pass, at an altitude of thirteen thousand feet (four thousand meters), connects Kullu Valley with Lahaul and

Spiti Valley. I slipped on stones and fell down a cliff, causing acute bleeding and nerve damage.

Three days later, my condition hadn't improved. Friends advised me to go to a Western-trained doctor at the hospital in Manali, the nearest town that was thirty-three miles (fifty-three kilometers) away. Apprehensive that a medical doctor would recommend surgery, I thought, "Why not go to the doctor of Tibetan medicine at the local Men-Tsee-Khang Clinic? I can find out if Tibetan medicine has an alternative option before subjecting myself to a surgery."

At the Men-Tsee-Khang Clinic, I remember vividly the look on the face of the resident doctor who happened to be a Tibetan Buddhist nun. She prescribed a seven-day course of Tibetan herbal medicines and said I would be fine. As she predicted, my symptoms disappeared in two days. The treatment's success completely intrigued me, giving me a newfound respect for Tibetan medicine and a deeper desire to become a doctor of Tibetan medicine. This experience made a lasting impression on me.

In 2003, I was in Manali again, this time to work on a book about Tibetan medicine. At the Men-Tsee-Khang Clinic, I asked to read the record book about my previous visit. I was curious to learn what Tibetan herbal medicines the doctor had prescribed that were so effective. According to the record, the doctor gave me three kinds of Tibetan medicines to stop the bleeding and repair my nerve damage. Since then, my fascination with Tibetan medicine has grown. For more than two decades, I have practiced Tibetan medicine and treated thousands of people across the globe with significant positive results.

Coming back to my initial meeting with Mim, Mike, and the students, we drove in an old bus through the foothills of Himalaya. We stayed at Swami Rama Sadhaka Grama Ashram near Rishikesh, India, and visited Himalayan Institute Hospital Trust and Ayurveda Center in Jolly Grant, India. Back on the bus, we drove sixteen hours to the Men-Tsee-Khang in Dharamsala, where Mim, Mike, and the students attended classes about Tibetan medicine. I taught the class about Men-Tsee-Khang research involving Tibetan medicines. Our group discovered and rediscovered these ancient wisdom traditions. Traveling and studying together was life transforming and humbling for each of us.

During this intellectual, spiritual journey, Mim and I discussed many topics involving Tibetan medicine. What excited us most was the possibility of collaborating on a book about Tibetan medicine. The following year in 2006, I again accompanied Mim and Mike, as well as a new group of University of Minnesota students. We traveled to the same sites as in 2005. While at Swami Rama Sadhaka Grama Ashram, Mim and I sat on the porch of a cottage and brainstormed about the book.

In the years to follow, both Mim and I found ourselves engaged with multiple projects that took us away from writing the book. However, the book was always part of our conversations. My second education demanded most of my time and energy. I decided to fulfill my dream of going to school in the United States. My goal was to study Western scientific methodology and conduct scientific research on Tibetan medicine.

Immigrating to the United States brought me much closer to Mim and Mike. At their suggestion, I applied to and was accepted at the University of Minnesota. They and their friends constantly were available to help me as I wrestled with my initial foray into Western-style education. During my four and a half years in Minnesota, Mim, Mike, and I sat at their kitchen table and engaged in thousands of hours of lively discussion. We talked about topics ranging from Tibetan medicine to philosophy to politics. This book, in many ways, results from those delightful, intellectually stimulating conversations.

The overarching strategy of this book is to present the complexity and rigorousness of Tibetan medicine in laypersons' language while maintaining the integrity of the fundamental teachings. Mim and I want to accomplish three main goals:

1. Share this ancient healing system with the wider population including health professionals, students, researchers, and everyone else.
2. Empower individuals to take charge of their own health by applying Tibetan medicine in everyday life.
3. Promote integrative care that includes Tibetan medicine.

These three goals are important, especially in our day and age where pluralistic health care has become a new norm. Individuals are exposed to and seek help from multiple health modalities. As many research studies have found, health approaches that complement each other provide more effective options than those that focus on only one perspective. Health professionals who want to provide informed, quality care need to develop understanding of diverse, effective healing traditions.

Recently, I conducted fieldwork in Tibetan refugee settlements in South India. These Tibetan refugees used Tibetan medicine along with Western medicines. They integrated Tibetan medicine with care from Western-trained doctors and nurses. However, I observed a lack of knowledge about Tibetan medicine among some of these health professionals. They didn't understand the mechanism and efficacy of Tibetan medicine. Hence, they created unnecessary conflict and a breakdown in crucial trust with the Tibetan refugees they were serving. Fortunately, I also encountered Tibetan health professionals trained in Western medicine who expressed genuine interest in learning about Tibetan medicine and its therapeutic potential. The book can be helpful for these health professionals.

Mim and I want to stimulate much-needed exchange of knowledge among health professionals in different disciplines. Moreover, we hope to encourage researchers to investigate Tibetan medicine. Most of all, our aspiration is for the book to help each reader create a happier, healthier, more conscious life.

In conclusion, I want to express my deep gratitude to Mim and Mike for helping me to accomplish my academic goals. I am grateful for our many personal and professional collaborations. I am also thankful to the Earl E. Bakken Center for Spirituality & Healing at the University of Minnesota for giving me an opportunity to teach and the Anthropology Department at Emory University for providing both funding and the intellectual milieu for my academic endeavors. However, I would be remiss not to express gratefulness to the Men-Tsee-Khang in Dharamsala, India, and all of my teachers at the Men-Tsee-Khang who paved the way for where I am today. I take immense pride in being a doctor of Tibetan medicine.

PART A

TIBETAN MEDICINE
AS SELF-CARE

How to Be Happy

$\mathcal{T}$ibetan medicine, the ancient yet timely science of healing from Tibet, teaches that everyone wants to be happy and to avoid suffering and dis-ease (lack of ease). This universal longing is elusive. All over the world, people are unhappy and suffering. You, too, may feel dissatisfied (lack of satisfaction). Tibetan medicine explains the complex relationship between mind, body, and environment, and why mind is the source of suffering. To be happy, you need to create a healthy mind.

Yes, you are affected by your genes, experiences, stress, emotions, thoughts, actions, age, health, diet, and environment. Your work, other people, microorganisms, money, politics, weather, and countless other variables influence you. When dealing with these factors, you are likely to make unhealthy choices if you don't know how to be happy. Poor choices lead to suffering and disease, rather than happiness and healing.

The first step toward happiness and healing is to behave ethically. Compassion is the most important ethical principle. However, an egotistic attitude, generated by the false belief in the existence of an intrinsic self, curtails ethical behavior and compassion.

You disturb your mind and body when you are violent toward yourself, others, and the environment by what you think, say, and do. The resulting imbalance creates suffering and illness. For example, negative self-talk, "I'm not good enough," fuels dissatisfaction and anger and depresses the immune system. Suffering and disease result from imbalance. Treating imbalance requires healing the source of the problem, not only the symptoms, and reestablishing balance.

The purpose of this chapter is to introduce Tibetan medicine's time-tested philosophy for creating, restoring, and sustaining health and happiness. Four complex, interrelated concepts underlie this profound tradition: karma, suffering, healing, and happiness. This chapter gives an overview of these concepts. Living according to these teachings won't create utopia but will help you to deal well with life's challenges and not make them worse. Subsequent chapters go into detail about application in everyday life.

KARMA

If everyone everywhere wants to be happy, why does the world have so much suffering? An answer is karma, the universal law of cause and effect. Karma, a Sanskrit term, means "As you sow, so shall you reap." For example, if you plant beans, you produce beans, not corn. Everything results from causes and has effects.

Similarly, the way to be happy is to make choices that lead to happiness rather than suffering. No matter what happens, deal wisely with each situation in a compassionate manner. You reap suffering if you plant suffering. To reap happiness, you need to plant happiness.

Theory of the Five Elements

To understand the influence of karma, you first must learn who you *really* are. You, like all phenomena, are composed of energy. This energy is called *joong-wa-nya*, a Tibetan word meaning the five sources of energy from which everything arises. These five sources are translated as five elements in English. Tibetans use a term from nature to describe each element. However, each element refers to a characteristic of energy, not specifically to **earth**, **water**, **fire**, **air**, and **space**.

All phenomena consist of the five elements (characteristics of energy):

- **Earth** provides stability and structure.
- **Water** produces moisture and smoothness.
- **Fire** drives growth, development, and absorption of food.
- **Air** governs movement in body and mind.
- **Space** allows the other elements to interact and coexist.

The **earth** element doesn't mean dirt. Instead, **earth** describes the characteristic of energy that gives stability and structure so that you can sit and stand. Unless you have sufficient **water** element, you will dry up and die. The **fire** element generates heat essential for digestion and metabolism. Because of the **air** element, you can move your body, your blood and lymph circulate, your organs function, and thoughts go through your mind. The **space** element makes room for the other four elements.

Theory of the Three Primary Energies

Earth, water, fire, and **air** interact to form three primary energies present in each living being:

1. *Loong* (**air**): movement energy (*vata* in Ayurveda, a traditional healing system from India).
2. *Tripa* (**fire**): hot energy (*yang* in Chinese medicine, *pitta* in Ayurveda).
3. *Baekan* (**water and earth**): cold energy (*yin* in Chinese medicine, *kapha* in Ayurveda).

The three primary energies are essential for life. *Loong* is pronounced loong. *Tripa* is pronounced teepa. *Baekan* is pronounced bacon. You, like everyone else, possess a unique combination of all three primary energies.

Loong energy, loosely translated as wind, regulates movement, both physical movement and thoughts in the mind. When thoughts are moving, the body is moving, and vice versa. *Loong* is related to *chi*, the term for life force in Chinese medicine, and *prana*, a Sanskrit term for life force in Ayurveda. Balanced *loong* can speed healing and aid in maintaining health and happiness. *Loong* is creative energy. Generally, writers, artists, musicians, actors, dancers, and other creative people have high *loong* energy.

Tripa energy, loosely translated as bile, is hot. *Tripa* controls heat in the body and mind and is responsible for metabolism, hunger, thirst, digestion, growth, and absorption of food and ideas. This hot energy promotes focus, clear thinking, courage, determination, goal setting, and achievement of goals. Ordinarily, leaders of all types have high *tripa*, and they set expectations for others.

Baekan energy, loosely translated as phlegm, is cold. **Baekan** maintains stability of the mind, as well as the structure, firmness, and smoothness of the body. This cold energy induces sleep, helps the body joints to function well, and lubricates the body. **Baekan** is the energy of patience and contentment.

You were born with a unique combination of these three primary energies, called *nyepa* in Tibetan. *Nyepa* literally means fault. If your state of balance is disrupted, the inherent nature of the *nyepa* is to cause harm to your well-being.

Your combination of the *nyepa* creates your true nature, your in-born constitutional nature, or simply your constitution. In the West, this blueprint is called your DNA or inherited genes. Your constitution, or home base, in large part determines your body shape, character, likes, dislikes, strengths, vulnerabilities, and ways of reacting and thinking. To *really* know yourself, you need to understand your constitution.

Theory of Seven Constitutions

Your constitution gets its name from its dominant energy or energies. For example, you have a **loong** constitution if **loong** dominates your **tripa** and **baekan**. Tibetan medicine describes seven general types of constitutions:

1. **Loong**: Movement energy dominates **tripa** and **baekan**.
2. **Tripa**: Hot energy dominates **loong** and **baekan**.
3. **Baekan**: Cold energy dominates **loong** and **tripa**.
4. **Loong/tripa** and **tripa/loong**: Movement and hot energies dominate **baekan**.
5. **Loong/baekan** and **baekan/loong**: Movement and cold energies dominate **tripa**.
6. **Tripa/baekan** and **baekan/tripa**: Hot and cold energies dominate **loong**.
7. **Loong/tripa/baekan** (rare constitution): All three energies are about equal.

Only highly evolved people are born with the ideal constitution: about equal percentages of *loong/tripa/baekan*. These individuals have ready access to all three primary energies. Keeping three equal energies in balance is complicated. Only highly evolved individuals are equipped to maintain this balance.

In most people, one or two primary energies dominate. For example, you have a *loong* constitution if your inborn energies are about 60 percent *loong*, 30 percent *tripa*, and 10 percent *baekan*. If your inborn constitution is made up of about 45 percent *loong*, 40 percent *tripa*, and 15 percent *baekan*, you have a *loong/tripa* constitution.

Knowing your constitution will help you to make healthy choices that keep the current percentages of your *nyepa* about the same as their percentages in your constitution. Through balanced living, you will enhance your strengths. You will transform your weaknesses into strengths, or at least keep them from sabotaging you.

Balance = Health; Imbalance = Dis-ease

Each of your three primary energies can be in a state of balance or out of balance, that is, rise too high, fall too low, and/or become disturbed. Similarly, when you boil water for tea, the water increases in volume as it gets hotter. If the water boils over or becomes steam, the volume of water decreases, and you may not have enough water for tea. Likewise, you are vulnerable to getting sick mentally and physically if any of your three energies rises too high, falls too low, and/or becomes disturbed.

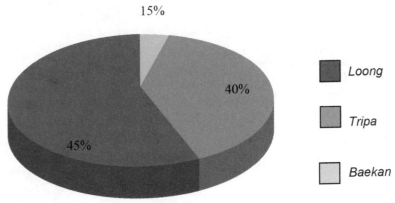

Example of a Loong-Tripa Constitution

Although your inborn constitution ordinarily doesn't change, conditions of life bombard your *nyepa*, requiring continual adjustment. Your diet, behavior, negativity, stress, genes, climate, stage in life, environment, and other variables disturb your *nyepa* and produce biochemical changes. Some regulation takes place automatically because of your internal wisdom, but other adjustment requires informed, mindful choices.

On the immediate level, health equals balance and disease equals imbalance of the three primary energies. The *nyepa* work together to produce mental and physical health. You are healthy when your current percentages of **loong**, **tripa**, and **baekan** are about the same as their percentages in your inborn constitution. Suffering and disease occur when they become too high, too low, and/or disturbed.

To be healthy and happy, you need to recognize when the current levels of your *nyepa* go out of balance with their levels in your constitution, and then take steps to reestablish equilibrium. Good choices produce balance, resulting in happiness and healing. Poor choices produce imbalance, resulting in suffering and disease. Because of karma, you become the person you create through your own choices.

SUFFERING

Suffering and Disease Begin in the Mind

Healing and happiness have a deeper dimension than the *nyepa*. Tibetan medicine teaches that healing and happiness begin in the mind. Because all phenomena are composed of energy, they are in a constant state of flux. Everything material is impermanent. Like all living beings, you are mortal and will die.

If you don't accept impermanence, you become attached to your ego. Self-centeredness leads to negative thinking, called mental poisons. Tibetan medicine describes three categories of mental poisons:

1. Greed, attachment, desire
2. Anger, hostility, aggression
3. Delusion, confusion, closed-mindedness

Mental poisons cloud your thinking. When under their influence, you likely will make unhealthy decisions about situations that confront you. Because of karma, poor choices produce suffering and disease, not healing and happiness.

The three mental poisons and resulting poor choices exert a devastating effect on your *nyepa*. Ordinarily, suffering and disease begin with *loong* imbalance. For example, you are anxious and can't sleep. Unless you correct this *loong* imbalance, your *tripa* and *baekan* likely will go out of balance, too. Imbalance in all three energies can produce complex, hard-to-unravel illnesses, such as cancer.

Tibetan medicine distinguishes between pain and suffering. For example, you may stumble, twist your ankle, and experience pain. You will suffer if you interpret your pain from a negative perspective, such as saying, "I'm a good person. Why doesn't life go well for me?" You can avoid suffering by letting go of negativity and saying, "Thankfully, I didn't break my ankle. This injury is telling me to slow down, and I'll do it."

Rather than say, "This is bad," or "This is good," simply say, "This is." Mindfully see the situation as it *really* is. Then figure out how best to deal with it. In this way, you will cope well with challenging situations and people instead of sabotaging yourself, disturbing your peace of mind, and even making things worse!

The true nature of the mind is like a cloudless sky. If you have a healthy mind, incidental obscurations pass by like clouds in the sky, and then the sky is clear again. You let go of negative thoughts, rather than compulsively think about them.

Obscurations occur because of negative karmic seeds planted in your mind, not because of what someone else does or what occurs. Eventually, these karmic seeds arise from their dormant state and appear, often unexpectedly. To be healthy and happy, you need to root out negative karmic seeds so that they no longer influence you.

When the three mental poisons are strong, obscurations conceal your pure, luminous mind, just as clouds block out the sun. This negativity interferes with your three primary energies and their sites in your mind and body. Understanding the relationship between the *nyepa* and three mental poisons is essential to transform this negativity into positive energy.

Relationship between the Three Primary Energies
and Three Mental Poisons

- **Loong** energy results from and leads to greed, attachment, and desire.
- **Tripa** energy results from and leads to anger, hostility, and aggression.
- **Baekan** energy results from and leads to delusion, confusion, and closed-mindedness.

*How **Loong** Is Related to Greed, Attachment, and Desire*

Loong imbalance causes and is caused by greed, (unhealthy) attachment, and desire. Dis-satisfaction (lack of satisfaction) is the source. Rather than create contentment, you want things to be different than they are. A childhood ditty illustrates this mental poison:

> I want what I want when I want it.
> I get what I want when I grab it.
> I get what I want, but don't want what I get.
> When I get what I want, I don't want it!

You feel anxious because you crave more, don't have what you want, or are afraid of losing what you do have. Rather than fulfill your needs, other people are more interested in meeting their own needs, which disappoints you. You are attracted to what you interpret to be pleasant and avoid what you think is unpleasant.

If you don't see things realistically, you fail to realize that what you interpret as pleasant may not be good for you and what you view as unpleasant may be beneficial for you. You don't understand the nature of attachment and aversion: They change continuously. You create a life of turmoil by being attached to what is impermanent.

Attraction and aversion induce tension in mind and body. Desire produces a restless mind and body, stress, nervousness, stiffness of neck and shoulders, and sleepless nights. Overthinking, brooding about the past, and constant worry about the future stir up *loong* energy. The mind becomes unstable and susceptible to external influences, like a flag fluttering in the wind. Mental turmoil weakens the mind and produces feelings of sadness, fear, and depression.

Too much, too little, and/or disturbed *loong* leads to movement disorders (lack of order) and aggravates existing imbalance. Anxious, you breathe in a shallow, rapid, irregular manner. Your cells don't become properly oxygenated and get rid of toxins. *Loong* imbalance causes stress-related problems: insomnia, nervousness, mood swings, heart palpitations, indigestion, irritable bowel syndrome, swirling thoughts, emotional distance, headaches, and depression. Chronic *loong* imbalance fosters mental illness and/or addiction to alcohol, drugs, food, relationships, sex, work, success, possessions, gambling, religion, and anything else.

When *loong* is out of balance, pressure builds, causing serious obstruction to blood flow. This imbalance negatively affects the heart. According to Tibetan medicine, subtle *loong* or mind resides in the heart and gut, not in the brain. The heart and gut take in sensations before the brain does. Channels carry these sensations to the brain, which in turn instructs the sense organs and body how to experience and deal with them. A heart attack and chronic intestinal problems can result from worrying about how to get what you want and avoid what you don't want.

When you feel depressed, notice your symptoms. They help you to learn about your constitution. You are more likely to develop *loong* depression if *loong* dominates your constitution. *Loong* depression is more serious if your dominant energy is *loong*. Similarly, if you have a *tripa* constitution you are more likely to develop *tripa* depression, and then *tripa* depression is graver for you. Likewise, you are vulnerable to *baekan* depression if you have a *baekan* constitution, and then *baekan* symptoms of depression are more serious for you.

Symptoms of **Loong**, **Tripa**, and **Baekan** Depression

- Loong depression: anxiety, insomnia, swirling thoughts, addictions.
- Tripa depression: anger, hostility, lashing out, aggression.
- Baekan depression: confusion, withdrawal, lethargy, procrastination.

How **Tripa** Is Related to Anger, Hostility, and Aggression

The second category of mental poisons is anger, hostility, and aggression. *Tripa* energy results from and is caused by this mental poison.

Tripa is hot and burns like a fire. When out of balance, ***tripa*** can inflame and destroy everything in its path. If you have a ***tripa*** constitution and/or your ***tripa*** is too high, you may try to do too much, lead a stressful life, and run over other people to get what you want.

Under the influence of this mental poison, you lack peace of mind and enjoyable relationships. Unhappy with life, you become irritable, antagonistic, and even hateful. Because you want to be successful, you get angry if anyone challenges or thwarts you. To save face, you are competitive, possessive, and hostile. You close yourself off from others and feel uneasy and depressed about how things are going.

As your isolation grows, your ego becomes all consuming, and you only see and hear yourself. You close the door to anything that doesn't fit into your categories. In your narrowing world, only two responses are possible: "I'm right!" and "They are wrong!" No longer do you engage in rational discussion with others because you think they are out to get you. You are "hot under the collar" about perpetual conflict in your life, and you explode with harsh behavior.

Too much heat can produce an elevated temperature, infections, inflammations, rapid pulse, headaches, rashes, metabolic and endocrine problems, digestive disorders, hot flashes, night sweats, and liver dysfunction. Your blood pressure rises, heart pounds, and face turns red. You perspire, and your perspiration smells foul. As with a *loong* imbalance, you breathe in a shallow, rapid, irregular manner. Your cells don't become properly oxygenated and let go of toxins. Anger, even justifiable anger, depresses your immune system. You may feel energized, but your mind is clouded, and you can't think clearly about how to deal well with your situation.

As your frustration grows, you abuse yourself, others, and the environment. Friends may suggest expressing anger. "Get it off your chest," they may advise. However, expressing anger or trying to hide anger causes problems. If you behave with anger and let anger eat away inside, your negative karma brings back harm to you.

How **Baekan** Is Related to Delusion, Confusion, and Closed-Mindedness

Baekan causes and is caused by delusion, confusion, and closed-mindedness. In a healthy state, ***baekan*** (cold energy) helps to keep ***tripa*** (hot energy) in balance. However, this mental poison causes **baekan** to rise in its diseased form. **Baekan** imbalance leads to cold disorders: you don't have enough heat. Instead, you have too much moisture and solidity. As a result, you are prone to developing laziness, procrastination, sleepiness, inertia, low metabolic rate, weak blood circulation, weight gain, obesity, diabetes, sinus congestion, colds, and edema.

As **baekan** increases, your digestive heat decreases. Your digestive system doesn't properly digest food. Even nutritious foods no longer nourish your body. Undigested particles of food accumulate and become toxic. Toxins clog your blood circulation and decrease oxygen to your brain and other organs.

An imbalance in cold energy originates from and creates a mind that is dull and lacking in awareness. A dazed, confused mind can't distinguish between virtue and vice, what is wise and what is unwise. Your ability to discriminate between right and wrong disappears. In such a bewildered state, you have difficulty understanding ideas, synthesizing them, arriving at conclusions, and making decisions

As you deny reality, you develop a judgmental attitude toward yourself and others. You don't learn from the past, integrate the present, and plan the future. Inevitably, you behave inappropriately and experience unfortunate results. You feel depressed because you lack understanding and insight.

The Three Primary Energies Affect Each Other

The *nyepa* are like a mobile over a baby's crib. When one primary energy goes out of balance, the other two primary energies are likely to become unbalanced, too. A similar mechanism occurs in the family. When one family member gets sick, the other members of the family are affected, too. Your **baekan** likely will decrease if your **tripa** rises too high. The opposite effect occurs when **baekan** rises too high.

When under the influence of the three mental poisons, you make poor choices. Yes, toxins, infectious diseases, other people, the environment, politics, your genes, weather, and many other factors influence you. Even so, you always have choices about how to deal with them. Healthy decisions promote balance, healing, and happiness. Poor choices produce imbalance that leads to suffering and disease.

HEALING

Goal of Healing: Health and Happiness

Healing results from rooting out the three mental poisons. When you no longer view your life from a negative perspective, you are able to behave virtuously and make choices that bring your *nyepa* back into balance with your constitution. You don't just treat symptoms, but you uncover and heal the source of your imbalance.

If, for example, you walk the wrong way, you may need to retrace your steps to walk in the direction you want to go. When knitting a sweater and you drop stitches, you may need to unravel the sweater to rectify the mistake. Without this correction, you could end up with a misshapen sweater. Similarly, you won't heal and be happy unless you uncover what is wrong in your life and make it right.

Happiness results from establishing harmony within yourself, with others, and with the universe. Live in a peaceful manner that is consistent with your constitution. First, though, you need to recognize when you are engaging in the three mental poisons. Then take steps to heal them by changing your thinking and behavior.

1. Greed, attachment, and desire: Result from and cause *loong* imbalance; meditate on and come to accept impermanence.
2. Anger, hostility, and aggression: Result from and cause *tripa* imbalance; meditate on and develop compassion.
3. Delusion, confusion, and closed-mindedness: Result from and cause *baekan* imbalance; meditate on and develop wisdom.

Heal Greed, Attachment, Desire, and **Loong** *Imbalance*

To heal greed, attachment, desire, and *loong* imbalance, meditate on and come to accept impermanence. All phenomena, including each of your cells, continuously change. Everything is interconnected and empty of inherent existence. Each phenomenon arises from and is dependent on other phenomena.

Impermanence means that all phenomena result from multiple causes and conditions. The individual you are now is an accumulation of all of your experiences. You change from moment to moment; you aren't the same person you were a moment ago, and you won't be the same individual a moment from now. And at the gross level, death is an obvious example of impermanence: You won't live forever.

To heal greed, attachment, desire, and *loong* imbalance, recognize that after meeting your basic needs impermanent phenomena won't make you happy. Train your mind to avoid craving what is material. You can't change the impermanent nature of things, including your body. Notice when you try to make permanent what is impermanent, such as a relationship, job, or anything else.

Heal greed, attachment, desire, and *loong* imbalance by dancing joyfully with the constant movement of life. Change what you can change and let go of everything else. Face impermanence with optimism and courage, rather than fear and sadness.

In addition to healing your thinking, you can calm *loong* energy by eating and drinking something warm, such as warm soup or herbal tea. If you are cold, put on a sweater. Avoid talking and be quiet. Do gentle yogic breathing and poses to be grounded. Walk in a nature center or go home and sit quietly. Do and think what is peaceful. Listen to soothing music. Still your mind.

Heal Anger, Hostility, Aggression, and **Tripa** *Imbalance*

You can heal anger, hostility, and aggression by meditating on and developing compassion. Compassion is the desire to relieve suffering for all living beings. Rather than a feeling, compassion is a philosophical stance of being kind to all people regardless of how they behave. Other individuals are of your own kind. They are made of the same five elements and *nyepa* that you are. Like you, they want to be happy and avoid suffering.

Compassion is not the same as caring. When you care for someone, you feel affection for the person. However, you may find it hard to care for enemies and strangers. You may even wish them ill! In contrast, compassion is an active, not passive, state of mind. Coming from a deep yearning, you ask, "What can I do to help?"

You can heal anger, hostility, and aggression by training your mind to deal well with challenging people and situations. They are your best teachers if you develop compassion. Discipline is needed to behave with compassion. You set appropriate limits to avoid being abused emotionally or physically. As you train your mind, you develop universal compassion, compassion toward all living beings, toward nature, and the universe.

Besides healing your thinking, you can cool your *tripa* energy by slowing down. Stop trying to do so much. Take time out when anger arises, rather than reacting right away. The situation isn't likely an emergency unless someone is bleeding profusely or can't breathe. After cooling down, you will think more clearly about how to deal with things in a manner that brings back good consequences, not poor ones.

To cool *tripa* energy, eat lightly cooked vegetables and stay away from spicy foods, alcohol, and other hot foods and beverages. Engage in cooling activities like walking in nature. Avoid vigorous exercise, such as jogging and hot yoga, that raises your temperature. Live and work in a peaceful, cool environment. Do gentle yogic breathing and poses.

Heal Delusion, Confusion, Closed-Mindedness and **Baekan** *Imbalance*

You can heal delusion, confusion, and closed-mindedness by meditating on and developing wisdom. Knowledge and wisdom are not the same. Knowledge consists of information and skills you acquire. Wisdom means to expand your consciousness and view things as they *really* are, based on your experiences and investigations, not as you want them to be. You see your situation in the context of the bigger picture.

Tibetan medicine teaches that wisdom means to be fully awake, as illustrated in this famous story about Shakyamuni Buddha, the historical Buddha.

A man asked the Buddha, "Who are you? Are you a god?"

"No," the Buddha said.

"Are you an angel?"

"No."

"Well, then, who are you?"

"I'm awake!" replied the Buddha.

Waking up means to take off blinders and colored glasses. If you go through life with only a partial view of things, you are likely to make poor lifestyle choices. Bring the contents of your unconscious mind into your consciousness mind. When you shine light on your unconscious mind, you will understand how and why you undermine yourself. Develop mindfulness each moment, and then you will be more likely to make healthy choices.

A woman rented a vacation house on a Greek island. When she drove up the mountain to the house, the weather was rainy and cloudy. She couldn't see the surrounding environment. The following morning, the rain stopped, and she could see a village on a mountain nearby. When she got up the next day, she not only could see the village but also the Mediterranean Sea far below. The following morning, the sky was so clear that she noticed islands in the Mediterranean. The next day, she could see the Greek mainland. As she opened the drapes the following day, she could see the spectacular, panoramic view of everything from the previous days, plus snow-topped mountains on the Greek mainland.

The next day, the weather was rainy and cloudy again. The woman couldn't see much beyond the house she was renting. However, this time she knew that the panoramic scene was still there. As illustrated by this story, wisdom is clear understanding that informs perception. When you are wise, you interpret your everyday experience according to your accurate comprehension of the way things *really* are.

Besides healing delusion, confusion, and closed-mindedness, you can warm **baekan** energy by exercising regularly. Walk fast, rather than slowly. Do yogic breathing and postures that cause your metabolism and heat to rise. If you are overweight, take off pounds so that your weight is appropriate. Overcome lethargy by adding stimulation. Don't procrastinate. Avoid napping during the day. Sip warm beverages. Eat warm, spicy foods. Live and work in a bright, dry, warm environment.

To develop wisdom, behave ethically in daily life and engage in spiritual practice. Mindfully choose what produces happiness, not suffering. Set up time for meditation each day. Through spiritual practice, you will develop a clearer mind.

As you develop wisdom, you realize why behaving ethically is vital for happiness. You make amends for hurting yourself, others, and the natural world. Instead of causing harm, you take every opportunity to do acts of loving-kindness. You make lifestyle choices that promote wholeness and peace so that you live a long, healthy, happy life and contribute to society.

Healing requires transforming intentions, not only thoughts and actions. Intentions become thoughts, thoughts turn into actions, actions develop into habits, and habits harden into character. Become fully conscious of your thoughts and make sure that they arise from kindly concern for everyone and everything.

Turmoil subsides as you transform the mental poisons into ethical behavior. Your mind quiets down. You heal in mind and body. Your mind heals, even if your body is not cured. Even on your deathbed, you can heal your mind and experience peace. Your *nyepa* become balanced with your constitution. You are happy.

HAPPINESS

Happiness means flourishing, self-actualization, excellence, well-being. You live with meaning, seeing your life as part of a bigger, meaningful picture. Behaving with integrity, you live according to your best values. The more you transform yourself, the happier you become. You develop optimal health, not simply an absence of disease.

When negative thoughts and feelings arise, you let them go and regain your balance. You train your mind to be wise, loving, compassionate, kind, honest, gentle, contented, responsible, altruistic, peaceful, nonviolent, joyful, patient, humble, tolerant, and forgiving. Perhaps forgiveness is the most difficult virtue to develop. You don't want to let off the hook the person who offended you.

The reason to forgive is so that you no longer carry the burden of resentment. Otherwise, you get hurt twice, first by the original event and second by how you react to it. Your negative reaction hurts you more and longer than the original event did. Forgiving doesn't mean to forget that the conflict occurred. Instead, forgiving is a process of transforming negativity into positive energy. By letting go of disappointment and hurt, you develop clearer thinking about how to deal with the situation in a manner that results in good consequences.

As you evolve ethically and spiritually, you create happiness and healing. You discover that you are linked with others, the natural world, and the universe. Mindful of karma, you realize that the energy you give out has a ripple effect. What you do affects others, and what they do affects you. Vowing to be loving-kindness, you reach out to help others and create a more compassionate, just world. Your inner wisdom and universal wisdom flow spontaneously through your mind and body.

SITTING MEDITATION AND CIRCULAR BREATHING

Meditation promotes this ethical, spiritual work. In Tibetan, meditation means to concentrate on something and become familiar with it. For instance, you can meditate on your mind to understand the nature of your mind. By focusing your attention, you calm your thoughts and develop mindfulness of reality. You begin to see things the way they *really* are, rather than as you want them to be. Getting to know your mind provides the opportunity to recognize and root out negative karmic seeds. You figure out why you cause suffering for yourself and others and transform this negativity into compassion and wisdom.

Tibetan medicine teaches that all actions are dependent on the mind. An unhealthy outlook produces unethical behavior and suffering. A mind that is not well controlled is likely to cause great harm. Therefore, the mind itself needs to be the principal object of meditation. Meditation serves to "tame" the mind, harmonize mind and body, and create a balanced state leading to inner and outer peace.

If you don't have much time to meditate, take two-minute breaks to focus on your breath and calm your mind. For example, excuse yourself from a meeting and go to the bathroom to meditate for two minutes. When you drive someplace, before getting out of your car, sit for two minutes and focus on your breath.

Meditation need not be mystical or otherworldly. You can meditate lying down, walking, standing, or sitting. If, however, you lie down to meditate, you may fall asleep. Walking while mediating may be distracting. You may not be able to meditate long if you stand up. Probably, you will focus best during Sitting Meditation.

How to Do Sitting Meditation and Circular Breathing

- Sit comfortably in a straight-back chair, on a meditation cushion, or on the floor.
- Straighten your back so that you can breathe deeply.
- Lower or close your eyes and relax your entire body.
- Breathe in a circular manner, through your nostrils, from your abdomen, slowly, deeply, evenly, with your in-breath the same length as your out-breath, and no break in between.

- As you inhale through your nose, silently count "One." Exhale. On the next in-breath, count, "Two," and so on.
- When your mind wanders, bring it back to your breath and start over with "One."
- If you reach "Ten," go back to "One."
- When you are deeply relaxed and focused, notice your inner experience. Simply observe and let go of whatever arises, without attachment, judgment, or direction.
- After your meditation, open your eyes and take this experience into your daily life.

After meditating, keep breathing in a circular manner. Circular breathing will help you to think clearly and your body to function smoothly. Your cells will take in life force and give off toxins. In time, you will train your mind to engage in circular breathing all the time. The mindfulness you develop through meditation will enhance your life.

You may experience difficulty sitting still and observing your mind. If so, do some yoga postures, take a walk, or engage in other exercise before meditating. After setting up a regular meditation practice, you gradually will be able to meditate for longer periods without distraction. Eventually, you will create a meditative mind-set while engaging in everyday activities.

In summary, Tibetan medicine's teachings about karma, suffering, healing, and happiness are life transforming. You will apply these teachings by setting up time to meditate each day and train your mind. As you become familiar with your mind, you will convert the three mental poisons into compassion and wisdom.

After reading this chapter, you probably are eager to learn about your own unique, inborn constitution composed of *loong*, *tripa*, and *baekan*. By coming to understand your constitution, you will choose what enhances your strengths and turns your weaknesses into strengths. The next chapter explains how to figure out your constitution and what choices are best for you.

· 2 ·

Live in Harmony with
Your Constitution

*T*ibetan medicine teaches that all phenomena consist of energy. *Joong-wa-nya* is the Tibetan term for the five energy sources from which everything arises. Tibetans use everyday words to describe them. *Sa*, translated as **earth**, means cold, structure, solidity. *Chu* or **water** is moisture, cohesion. *Mey* or **fire**, means heat. *Loong*, translated as air, is movement. *Namkha* or space allows the other four energy sources to coexist and interact. The five energy sources, called elements, are essential for all existence.

The five elements interact to form three primary energies: (1) *loong*, movement energy; (2) *tripa*, hot energy; and (3) *baekan*, cold energy. They are called *nyepa*, a Tibetan word for fault. *Loong*, *tripa*, and *baekan* are crucial for life but become faults if they go out of balance and transform into sources of disease.

Like everyone, you were born with a unique combination of the five elements and three *nyepa*. Your blend of the *nyepa* is called your true nature, constitutional nature or, simply, constitution. In conventional health care, the blueprint you are born with is called your DNA or inherited genes. Your inborn constitution, or home base, largely determines your body shape, character, likes, dislikes, strengths, weaknesses, and ways of thinking. To create health and happiness, you need to live in harmony with your constitution.

This chapter explains two research-based, self-assessment tools based on Tibetan medicine that will help you to learn about your constitution and lifestyle choices that are best for you. You can complete these tools on your own or, ideally, use them in combination with a consultation by an experienced, qualified Tibetan medicine doctor, in the United States called a Tibetan medicine practitioner. The chapter ends with a meditation on the lotus flower, an inspiring symbol of beauty and transformation.

GOLD STANDARD: CONSULTATION WITH A TIBETAN MEDICINE PRACTITIONER

Tibetan medicine offers an ancient, timely, holistic model for promoting health and treating disease by encouraging healthy decisions. You learn about your unique inborn constitution. Then you make choices to support your constitution and create a happier, healthier life. Ideally, you heal the source of imbalance, not just symptoms.

A healthy mind is essential to make choices that keep your *nyepa* in harmony with your constitution. You are healthy when the current percentages of your *loong*, *tripa*, and *baekan* are about the same percentages as in your inborn constitution. By living a balanced life, you learn to enhance your strengths and turn your weaknesses into strengths, or at least keep them from being a negative influence.

A qualified, experienced Tibetan medicine practitioner is the gold standard for constitutional analysis. First, she or he observes you, analyzes your urine, looks at your tongue, reads your radial pulses, and asks you questions. Next, the practitioner diagnoses your constitution and what, if any, energies are out of balance. Finally, the person prescribes lifestyle choices that support your constitution, as described in this book.

You will need at least three consultations to identify your constitution and determine if your *nyepa* are in balance. Ordinarily, your constitution doesn't change. However, your *loong*, *tripa*, and *baekan* can rise too high, fall too low, or become disturbed depending on what is going on in your life. If the current state of your *nyepa* is not consistent with your constitution, the practitioner may have difficulty identifying your constitution. Several consultations over time help the practitioner make an accurate assessment.

Before scheduling a consultation, inquire about the practitioner's credentials. Select someone who graduated from a qualified Tibetan medical college. Currently, education to practice Tibetan medicine is not standardized and ranges from apprenticeships to five or more years of medical education plus one or more years of internship supervised by senior practitioners. Moreover, find out if the person is experienced in constitutional assessment and pulse diagnosis. Without an excellent medical education and experience, the practitioner may not give you correct information. Go to chapter 13 for details about a Tibetan medicine consultation.

Besides consulting with an experienced, qualified Tibetan medicine practitioner, you can learn about your constitution by completing the Constitutional Self-Assessment Tool (CSAT). Using your CSAT results, complete the Lifestyle Guidelines Tool (LGT) and create a plan for living in harmony with your constitution. These research-based tools do not substitute for an experienced practitioner. However, they provide insight about your constitution and lifestyle choices to help you to create health and happiness.

CONSTITUTIONAL SELF-ASSESSMENT TOOL AND LIFESTYLE GUIDELINES TOOL

Research-Based Self-Assessment Tools

We created the Constitutional Self-Assessment Tool (CSAT) to help our students identify their constitution. After completing the CSAT, the students requested guidelines about living in harmony with their constitution. We then created the Lifestyle Guidelines Tool (LGT). Both tools are based on the *Gyueshi*, the fundamental text of Tibetan medicine. We wrote each CSAT and LGT item to be authentic to the *Gyueshi*, understandable in English, and applicable in everyday life.

Next, we organized a research team to test the content and criterion validity of and to refine the CSAT and LGT. The study was funded by a competitive grant from the University of Minnesota's Earl E. Bakken Center for Spirituality & Healing. Content validity means that the CSAT and LGT are based on Tibetan medicine, as described in the *Gyueshi*. Criterion validity means that the CSAT correctly identifies one's dominant energy at the time of the assessment, as described in *Gyueshi*. Our research team used a mixed methods design (quantitative and qualitative) and met all the requirements for protection of human subjects.

Phase One: Investigate Content Validity of the CSAT and LGT   Cameron met twice with six experienced, senior Tibetan medicine practitioners at the Men-Tsee-Khang Tibetan Medical College in Dharamsala, India. The purpose was to evaluate the content validity of the CSAT and LGT. All six evaluators answered three questions about each item in the tools: (1) How relevant is this item to Tibetan medicine? (2) Is this item clearly written? (3) What, if any, items about Tibetan medicine are needed that we failed to include?

The evaluators and Cameron refined each item of the CSAT and LGT. At the end of both meetings, all six evaluators (100 percent) agreed that the tools accurately portray Tibetan medicine as described in the *Gyueshi*. As a result, the CSAT and LGT have high content validity.

Phase Two: Investigate Criterion Validity of the CSAT   The research participants consisted of fifty-nine adult students at a university in the United States who had not studied Tibetan medicine. Their mean age was thirty-three; 83 percent were female; 90 percent were Caucasian, and 10 percent were other ethnicities. Each student had a forty-five-minute confidential consultation with Namdul, a qualified, experienced Tibetan medicine practitioner. Namdul filled out a form with information about the student's constitution and optimal choices. After reading the form, the student completed the LGT and answered five questions about the CSAT and LGT:

1. What did you like about completing the CSAT? The LGT?
2. What didn't you like about completing the CSAT? The LGT?
3. Are the tools helpful for you? Why or why not?
4. What suggestions do you have for improving the tools?
5. Do you have any other feedback for us?

Next, we recruited students at the university who had attended at least nine hours of a graduate course about Tibetan medicine. The twenty-nine students followed a modified Phase Two method. Their mean age was thirty-five, 86 percent were female, and 100 percent were Caucasian. Each student completed the CSAT, had a confidential consultation with Namdul, completed the LGT, and wrote answers to the same five questions.

We compared each student's CSAT result with the gold standard: Namdul's constitutional assessment of the student. Then we compared all of the students' CSAT results with Namdul's assessments of all of the students. Using more than one Tibetan medicine practitioner was beyond the scope of this study.

For the students who had not studied Tibetan medicine, the CSAT had 51 percent agreement and .24 kappa statistic, suggesting fair criterion validity of the CSAT. Students who had studied Tibetan medicine completed the refined CSAT with a 76 percent agreement and .50 kappa statistic. These results suggest moderate criterion validity of the CSAT. Criterion validity improved if students knew basic teachings of Tibetan medicine and did accurate self-assessments.

Phase Three: Refine the CSAT and LGT   Finally, we employed Cameron's published phenomenological method[1] to analyze the students' answers to the five qualitative questions. Cameron and her colleagues had used this method in several studies. All of the students in both groups wrote enthusiastically about completing the CSAT and LGT together. For them, the CSAT alone was insufficient if they did not know what lifestyle choices were best.

Five themes emerged from the students' statements about CSAT benefits. These themes were (1) information about a student's constitution, (2) surprise about what is relevant for health and happiness, (3) self-understanding, (4) self-improvement, and (5) a new perspective. As one student put it, "The CSAT helped me to realize how I push myself to be different than what I naturally am and to nurture the parts of me I tend to dislike." Another student wrote, "The CSAT raised my awareness of patterns in my life that may contribute to imbalance."

Five themes became apparent in the students' statements about LGT benefits. These themes were (1) information about how to create balance, (2) surprise about what lifestyle choices are best, (3) self-understanding, (4) self-improvement, and (5) confirmation about "what I can do." As one student wrote, "The LGT shows that I do know myself better than I thought and what I should do in the future."

Three themes emerged from the students' statements about the challenge of completing the two tools. They were (1) choosing only one option per CSAT characteristic, (2) self-reporting, and (3) resistance. Most students had difficulty assessing themselves accurately. A student asked, "What is my normal?" Some students resisted the LGT because it "forced me to confront negative aspects of myself and consider changes that I do not want to make."

Throughout the research process, we used the quantitative and qualitative findings to refine the CSAT and LGT. We edited the wording of items to improve distribution, tone, clarity, and applicability. In each subsequent draft, the content and format remained the same as in the original CSAT and LGT validated by the six senior practitioners of Tibetan medicine.

We published the research, along with the CSAT and LGT.[2] In addition, the CSAT and LGT are available online for free, confidential use 24/7.[3] Since we conducted the study, nearly one thousand diverse students have taken our graduate courses about Tibetan medicine at the University of Minnesota.[4] All the students wrote papers about their experience of completing the CSAT and LGT. The students' papers support these research findings.

COMPLETE THE CONSTITUTIONAL SELF-ASSESSMENT TOOL (CSAT)

Go ahead and complete the CSAT below. The CSAT will help you to learn about Tibetan medicine and apply the teachings in your life. Do the CSAT again and again. Each time, you will understand better the importance of the items and how they affect your health and happiness.

Information to Help You Fill Out the CSAT Accurately

What is the CSAT?
The CSAT is based on Tibetan medicine, an ancient, timely, holistic healing system from Tibet. Tibetan medicine teaches that you, like everyone else, were born with a unique nature, called your constitution. The CSAT will help you to understand your own constitution.

What Do You Mean by My Constitution?
Your constitution is your unique combination of three primary, essential energies:

1. *Loong* (pronounced loong)—movement energy
2. *Tripa* (pronounced teepa)—hot energy
3. *Baekan* (pronounced bacon)—cold energy

How Is My Constitution Made Up of the Three Primary Energies?
The name of your constitution comes from your primary energy. For example, your constitution may be about 80 percent *tripa*, 15 percent *baekan*, and 5 percent *loong*. Therefore, you have a *tripa* constitution. However, you have a dual constitution if two energies dominate. For example, you have a *tripa/baekan* constitution if you have about 45 percent *tripa*, 35 percent *baekan*, and 20 percent *loong*.

What Are the Seven Constitutions of Tibetan Medicine?

1. *Loong*
2. *Tripa*
3. *Baekan*
4. *Loong/tripa* and *tripa/loong*
5. *Loong/baekan* and *baekan/loong*
6. *Tripa/baekan* and *baekan/tripa*
7. *Loong/tripa/baekan* (Only highly-evolved individuals are born with this rare constitution.)

Does My Constitution Change throughout My Life?
No, but your primary energies can increase, decrease, and/or become disturbed because of your thoughts, lifestyle choices, and situation. If, for example, your constitution is about 40 percent *tripa*, you have too much *tripa* if it goes above 40 percent, and you have too little *tripa* if it goes below 40 percent. To be healthy and happy, you need to make lifestyle choices that bring your three primary energies back to their percentages in your constitution.

How to Complete the CSAT

Complete the CSAT to identify which of your three primary energies (*loong*, *tripa*, or *baekan*) dominates your constitution. Follow these nine steps:

1. For each characteristic, write only **one X in either the *loong*, *tripa*, or *baekan* column**
2. Select the description that describes who you *really* are, not the person you want to be.
3. Select the one description of *loong*, *tripa*, or *baekan* that best describes you, even if you don't fit this description completely or you fit into more than one description.
4. Assess yourself accurately; feel free to consult with someone who knows you well.
5. Take time to complete the CSAT.
6. Redo your answers if you don't think they are accurate.
7. Count the number of times you wrote X in each column and put the total in the box at the bottom of the column.
8. Add the totals of all three columns to make sure that they = 47, if you included #14 (menstruation). Otherwise, your overall total should = 46.
9. Redo the CSAT if your three scores are nearly equal.

How to Figure Out Your Dominant Primary Energy

Determine which column has the highest score, the second highest score, and the third highest score. The column with the highest score is your dominant primary energy. If your assessment is accurate, this energy gives the name to your constitution. For example, you have a *tripa* constitution if *tripa* is higher than your other two primary energies.

Two primary energies may dominate your third energy. If your assessment is accurate, you have a dual constitution. For example, you have a *tripa/baekan* constitution if *tripa* and *baekan* dominate *loong*.

If your *nyepa* are out of balance, you likely will have difficulty identifying your constitution. Ideally, the CSAT will identify your primary energy that currently is dominant. This result may differ from your actual dominant primary energy in your constitution. If, for example, you are stressed out, *loong* may be your CSAT dominant primary energy, even though you have a *tripa* or *tripa-baekan* constitution. The LGT can help you to bring the current percentages of your three primary energies back to their percentages in your constitution.

Constitutional Self Assessment Tool (CSAT)

	Characteristics	Loong		Tripa		Baekan	
1	My height is:	☐	Short, or unusually tall; slightly stooped posture.	☐	Average.	☐	Above average; erect posture.
2	My weight is:	☐	Tendency to be underweight; hard to gain, easy to lose.	☐	Average, with minor fluctuations; easy to gain and lose.	☐	Tendency to be overweight; easy to gain, hard to lose.
3	My body frame is:	☐	Thin, light.	☐	Muscular, proportional.	☐	Strong, stocky.
4	My skin tends to be:	☐	Dry, rough	☐	Warm, oily.	☐	Cool, smooth.
5	When exposed to the sun, my skin:	☐	Tans without sunburn.	☐	Becomes red and rarely tans.	☐	Darkens after a mild sunburn.
6	My hair naturally tends to be:	☐	Dry, coarse, curly; prone to dandruff and split ends.	☐	Fine, straight; prone to premature graying and baldness.	☐	Thick, wavy, healthy, lustrous.
7	My eyes tend to be:	☐	Dry.	☐	Prone to redness and irritation.	☐	Well-lubricated.
8	My joints tend to be:	☐	Stiff with cracking sounds.	☐	Flexible.	☐	Well-lubricated with few cracking sounds.
9	My nails are:	☐	Thin, brittle.	☐	Soft, smooth.	☐	Strong, thick.
10	My skin tends to be:	☐	Prone to chapping, corns, calluses, cracked heels.	☐	Sensitive; prone to acne, rashes, freckles, moles.	☐	Moist, not prone to skin irritations.
11	My teeth are:	☐	Sensitive, uneven; gums may recede early.	☐	Prone to cavities, bleeding gums, canker sores.	☐	Even, large, strong.
12	My appetite is:	☐	Irregular, ranging from hunger to a lack of appetite.	☐	Excellent, but I become irritable without regular meals.	☐	Moderate; I love sweets and am prone to emotional snacking.
13	My digestive heat (metabolic rate) is:	☐	Fluctuating; my digestion varies from fast to slow.	☐	High; I digest food fast.	☐	Low; I digest food slowly.
14	My menstruation, without medication, is (if applicable):	☐	Irregular, scanty; PMS: anxiety, insomnia, moodiness.	☐	Regular; PMS: irritability, rashes, headaches, cravings.	☐	Long duration, heavy; PMS: cramping, bloating, lethargy.
15	My blood circulation is:	☐	Irregular; my body temperature varies from cold to hot.	☐	Good; I feel warm, and my hands and feet are warm.	☐	Weak; I feel cold, and often have cold hands and feet.
16	My bowel movements tend to be:	☐	Irregular, periodic constipation.	☐	Frequent, loose.	☐	Regular, formed.
17	Throughout my life, I have been:	☐	Free spirited.	☐	Goal-oriented.	☐	Easy-going.
18	My sweat is:	☐	Minimal.	☐	Plentiful.	☐	Moderate.
19	My voice tends to:	☐	Vary in volume, be prone to hoarseness.	☐	Be loud, distinct.	☐	Be low, soft.
20	My energy level is:	☐	Variable.	☐	High.	☐	Steady.
21	I tend to engage in this kind of exercise:	☐	Vigorous exercise, but I quickly get exhausted.	☐	Vigorous exercise, which refreshes me.	☐	Mild, if any, exercise.
22	My sleep is:	☐	Light, irregular.	☐	Good, but irregular at times.	☐	Deep, long.
23	My sex drive is:	☐	Variable, with active fantasy life.	☐	High, with passionate desire.	☐	Moderate, with slow arousal.
24	I'm susceptible to this combination of symptoms:	☐	Insomnia, anxiety, ringing in ears, shifting pain.	☐	Fever, infection, acid reflux, nausea.	☐	Colds, water retention, weight gain, slow digestion.
25	When stressed out, I tend to be:	☐	Fearful, insecure, tense.	☐	Angry, judgmental, irritable.	☐	Complacent, inflexible, procrastinating.
26	My personality tends to be:	☐	Lively, creative, flexible, enthusiastic, sensitive.	☐	Ambitious, competitive, goal-directed, motivated, adventurous.	☐	Calm, persistent, considerate, serious, humble.

#						
27	When upset, I tend to be:	☐	Anxious, restless, indecisive.	☐	Demanding, frustrated, hot-tempered.	☐ Withdrawn, inactive, resentful.
28	My dreams when I sleep tend to be:	☐	Busy, incoherent.	☐	Adventurous, intense.	☐ Coherent, calm.
29	My learning style is:	☐	Variable, unfocused.	☐	Quick, focused.	☐ Relaxed, steady.
30	My speech is:	☐	Excited, talkative, jumping from topic to topic.	☐	Convincing, confident, argumentative.	☐ Pleasant, deliberate, not talkative.
31	My approach to work is:	☐	Imaginative, original; I have many ideas but lack focus to carry them out.	☐	Methodical, focused; I enjoy developing and then delegating new projects.	☐ Practical, managerial; I am less able to initiate a new project, but I can make it run smoothly.
32	I am happiest when I am:	☐	With a group of people, talking, laughing, singing, dancing.	☐	With friends engaging in competitive, adventurous activities.	☐ Having a quiet, comfortable time alone or with a few good friends.
33	In dealing with other people, I tend to be:	☐	Excited, imaginative.	☐	Courageous, determined.	☐ Loving, compassionate.
34	I tend to have this negativity:	☐	Greed, desire.	☐	Anger, hostility.	☐ Confusion, closed-mindedness.
35	I learn:	☐	Easily, but I quickly forget.	☐	Easily, and I remember what I learn.	☐ Methodically, and I apply learning for a long time.
36	My confidence level is:	☐	Low; I lack confidence on the surface and inside.	☐	High on the surface, but I lack confidence inside.	☐ Low on the surface, but I have inner confidence.
37	My mind tends to be:	☐	Restless.	☐	Goal-directed.	☐ Satisfied.
38	My veins are:	☐	Highly visible.	☐	Visible.	☐ Faintly visible.
39	To relax, I:	☐	Socialize, engage in artistic activities.	☐	Exercise, engage in competitive activities.	☐ Read, engage in quiet activities.
40	My friendships are characterized by:	☐	I know many people; my friendships are brief and lack closeness.	☐	I make friends easily and have many good friends.	☐ I slowly make friends, and develop lasting friendships with a few people.
41	Typically I react in this way to change:	☐	Anxious, flexible.	☐	Reactive, direct.	☐ Resistant to change, cautious.
42	I enjoy this combination of foods and beverages:	☐	Salads, soups, coffee, energy drinks.	☐	Spicy foods, French fries, meat, alcohol.	☐ Sweets, snacks, starchy foods, fruit juices.
43	My spending habits tend to be:	☐	Spontaneous.	☐	Sensible.	☐ Frugal.
44	When I experience pain, I tend to be:	☐	Hypersensitive.	☐	Impatient.	☐ Withdrawn.
45	I prefer this climate:	☐	Hot, humid.	☐	Cool, dry.	☐ Warm, dry.
46	My lifestyle is:	☐	Unplanned.	☐	Organized.	☐ Stable.
47	Here is how I tend to approach life:	☐	Question and doubt.	☐	Strive to get ahead.	☐ Be content.
	Total Xs in each column:					
	For %, divide each total by 47 (46 if #14 is NA):					
	My dominant energy:					
	Date of assessment:					

COMPLETE THE LIFESTYLE GUIDELINES TOOL

Using your CSAT result, complete the LGT below. The LGT will help you to learn about Tibetan medicine and create a plan to live in harmony with your constitution. Do the CSAT and LGT regularly. Each time you complete the tools, you will understand better the importance of the items and how they affect your happiness and health.

Information to Help You Fill Out the LGT Accurately

What Is the LGT?

The Lifestyle Guidelines Tool (LGT) and Constitutional Self-Assessment Tool (CSAT) are based on Tibetan medicine. Use them together to develop a personalized plan for living a healthier, happier life.

How to Complete the LGT

Complete the CSAT to identify which of your three primary energies (*loong, tripa,* or *baekan*) dominates your constitution. Follow these nine steps to complete the LGT:

1. On the LGT, write your CSAT result and the date you complete the LGT.
2. Follow the column of the LGT with the same name as your CSAT dominant primary energy. For example, follow the *tripa* column if *tripa* is your dominant primary energy. *If you have a dual constitution, follow both columns of your two dominant primary energies. For example, follow both the loong and tripa columns to calm loong and cool tripa.*
3. Check the small boxes of the large boxes in this column to indicate which guidelines you are willing and able to incorporate into your life now.
4. Develop a personalized plan for applying the guidelines you checked.
5. Prioritize your checked guidelines.
6. Select the three guidelines with the highest priority.
7. Write these three guidelines at the bottom of the LGT and explain how you will apply them.

8. Apply these three guidelines in your life.
9. When you are ready, apply the other prioritized guidelines in your life.

Periodically, complete the CSAT and LGT and develop a new plan. You will learn how to reestablish balance and maximize your health and happiness.

USE THE CONSTITUTIONAL SELF-ASSESSMENT TOOL AND LIFESTYLE GUIDELINES TOOL TOGETHER

How to Use the Tools Together

The research results lend support for using the CSAT and LGT together to bring your *nyepa* back into harmony with your constitution and to maintain balance. First, complete the CSAT to identify your dominant primary energy at the time of doing the CSAT. Ideally, this result is the dominant primary energy in your inborn constitution. Then, follow the LGT column of your dominant primary energy to make healthy lifestyle choices.

If, for example, you complete the CSAT and find that *loong* is your dominant primary energy, then follow the LGT column for *loong* to calm your *loong*. The LGT *tripa* column cools *tripa*. The LGT *baekan* column warms *baekan*. You may have a dual constitution. Then follow both LGT columns of your two dominant energies. For example, follow both the *tripa* and *baekan* columns to cool *tripa* and warm *baekan*.

The LGT has space for you to develop a personalized plan for healthy living. If you try to make too many changes at once, you probably will fail. Therefore, the LGT offers a practical approach. Prioritize the LGT items and list your top three priorities. Then answer for each priority, "How I will apply this guideline in my life."

Periodic evaluations will indicate when you are out of balance. For example, the CSAT may indicate that *loong* is your dominant primary energy, although you have a *tripa* constitution. If so, follow the LGT *loong* column to calm *loong*. If your next CSAT result shows *baekan* to be dominant, follow the LGT *baekan* column to warm *baekan*. The

LIFESTYLE GUIDELINES TOOL (LGT)

My CSAT dominant energy: _____   Date of completing LGT: _____

	Lifestyle choices:	*Loong* (Calms Loong)	*Tripa* (CoolsTripa)	*Baekan* (Warms Baekan)
1	Meals:	☐ Regular meals with moderate amounts of food, beverages; avoid skipping meals.	☐ Regular meals with moderate amounts of food, beverages; eat on time.	☐ Regular meals with moderate amounts of food, beverages; avoid snacking, overeating.
2	Foods and beverages:	☐ Warm, cooked foods and beverages that are, if possible, organic, fresh, natural, and locally grown.	☐ Warm, cooked foods and beverages that are, if possible, organic, fresh, natural, and locally grown.	☐ Warm, cooked foods and beverages that are, if possible, organic, fresh, natural, and locally grown.
3	Lean meat (for meat eaters):	☐ Beef, lamb, chicken, turkey, seafood.	☐ Pork, goat.	☐ Lamb, chicken, turkey, fish.
4	Spices and herbs:	☐ Caraway, cardamom, chives, cinnamon, cloves, coriander, cumin, garlic, fresh ginger, mustard, nutmeg, parsley, pepper.	☐ Cilantro, cumin, mint, parsley, saffron, turmeric.	☐ Caraway, cardamom, chives, cinnamon, cloves, coriander, cumin, garlic, dried ginger, mustard, nutmeg, parsley, pepper.
5	Cooked vegetables:	☐ Asparagus, beets, broccoli, corn, carrots, fennel, green beans, leeks, mushrooms, onions, peas, radish, red cabbage, seaweed, sweet potatoes, tomato, turnip, yam, zucchini.	☐ Beets, broccoli, cabbage, cauliflower, carrots, celery, cucumbers, eggplant, green beans, leafy greens, mushrooms, okra, peas, potatoes, pumpkin, rhubarb, seaweed, squash, sweet pepper, tomato, yam, zucchini.	☐ Asparagus, beets, carrots, fennel, garlic, green beans, hot peppers, leeks, onions, radish, seaweed, spinach, tomato, turnip, zucchini.
6	Naturally derived sweeteners:	☐ Molasses.	☐ Raw sugar.	☐ Honey.
7	Nuts and seeds:	☐ Moderate amounts.	☐ Small amounts.	☐ Moderate amounts.
8	Grains:	☐ All grains in moderation; minimal amounts of refined rice and flour.	☐ All grains in moderation; minimal amounts of refined rice and flour.	☐ All grains in moderation; minimal amounts of refined rice and flour.
9	Fruits:	☐ Apples, apricots, avocados, bananas, berries, coconut, fresh figs, grapes, grapefruit, peaches, melon, mango, oranges, papaya, pears, pineapple, plums, prunes.	☐ Apples, avocado, coconut, dates, fresh figs, grapes, mango, melon, oranges, pears, pineapples, plums, pomegranate, prunes, raisins.	☐ Apples, apricots, berries, cranberries, dry figs, lemons, mango, oranges, papaya, peaches, pears, persimmon, pomegranate, prunes, raisins.
10	Dairy products (if tolerated):	☐ More dairy products.	☐ Moderate dairy products.	☐ Less dairy products.
11	Legumes (e.g. beans, lentils, peas):	☐ Moderate amounts of legumes.	☐ More legumes.	☐ Less legumes.
12	Oils:	☐ More oils.	☐ Moderate amounts.	☐ Less oils.
13	Tastes to savor:	☐ Salty, sour, sweet.	☐ Astringent (e.g. avocado, raw banana, black tea), bitter, sweet.	☐ Hot (spicy), salty, sour.
14	Tastes to avoid:	☐ Astringent (e.g. avocado, raw banana, black tea), bitter.	☐ Hot (spicy), salty, sour.	☐ Astringent (e.g. avocado, raw banana, black tea), bitter, sweet.

15	Sleep:	☐ Sound and regular.	☐ Sound and regular.	☐ Sound and regular.
16	Sex (if applicable):	☐ Less sex.	☐ Moderate sex.	☐ More sex.
17	Vacation:	☐ Calming time with a few close friends.	☐ Relaxing time, without disturbance.	☐ Active, stimulating time.
18	Mental state:	☐ Calm, soothing, grounded.	☐ Cool, relaxing, non-competitive.	☐ Warm, stimulating, social.
19	Environment:	☐ Warm, humid.	☐ Cool, dry.	☐ Warm, dry.
20	Environment to avoid:	☐ Cold, dry.	☐ Hot, humid.	☐ Cold, humid.
21	Physical activities:	☐ Light, regular exercise, including walking, gentle yoga.	☐ Moderate, regular exercise, including brisk walking, gentle yoga.	☐ Vigorous, regular exercise, including jogging, active yoga.
22	Physical activities to avoid:	☐ Exercising on an empty stomach.	☐ Engaging in vigorous activities in a hot environment.	☐ Not exercising and excercising sporadically.
23	Behaviors to avoid:	☐ Talking too much, watching upsetting shows, playing disturbing video games.	☐ Confrontation, sleeping during the day in hot weather, taking a sauna or steam bath.	☐ Overeating; sleeping right after eating; sleeping in a damp, cool environment.
24	Attitudes to avoid:	☐ Greed, attachment, desire.	☐ Anger, hostility, aggression.	☐ Confusion, delusion, closed-mindedness.
25	Meditation:	☐ Accept impermanence.	☐ Develop compassion.	☐ Develop wisdom.

My personalized plan:

Priority #1:	How I will apply this guideline in my life:
Priority #2	How I will apply this guideline in my life:
Priority #3	How I will apply this guideline in my life:

CSAT can help you to bring your *nyepa* back to their percentages in your constitution.

By regularly completing the CSAT and LGT, you will learn about your *loong*, *tripa*, and *baekan* and how to keep them in sync with your constitution. Ideally, you will identify and reverse imbalance before you get sick. As Tibetan medicine teaches, dance through life and continually reestablish balance.

Do Accurate CSAT Assessments

Studies have been published about the challenges of doing accurate self-assessments. When completing the CSAT, assessing yourself correctly is essential. For example, you may have a *tripa* constitution. However, you are likely to overreport *loong* if you are stressed-out, tired, and hungry, and you make lifestyle choices that aggravate *loong*. Then your CSAT result likely will be *loong*, rather than *tripa*.

Some students who participated in the research were anxious because of school, work, debt, relationships, and other issues. They had too many deadlines, lack of sleep, too much coffee, and not enough money. These students tended to overreport *loong*. Consequently, their CSAT result was *loong* because their *loong* was elevated when they took the CSAT. When doing these students' assessments, Namdul often identified *tripa* or *baekan*, not *loong*, as the dominant primary energy in the student's constitution. The students' CSAT results that did not correspond with Namdul's assessments lowered the criterion validity of the CSAT.

Like the students, you may overreport *loong* if you are stressed-out and your *loong* is elevated. Moreover, you may score too high on *tripa* if you do the CSAT when you are agitated and angry. During the cold of winter, you may overreport *baekan*. Wait to complete the CSAT until you have calmed down, cooled off, or warmed up.

The research sheds light on how to increase the accuracy of your CSAT result. The findings suggest that students who had studied Tibetan medicine before completing the CSAT did more accurate CSAT assessments than students who didn't know much, if anything, about Tibetan medicine. Students with some knowledge of Tibetan medicine understood the CSAT items better than did students new to Tibetan medicine.

How to Increase Accuracy of Your CSAT Result

- Learn about Tibetan medicine to help you understand the CSAT items.
- Complete the CSAT when you are feeling "like yourself," not when you are hungry, anxious, angry, late, tired, or confused.
- Complete the CSAT in a quiet, comfortable environment, without time pressures.
- Do the CSAT with someone who knows you well, such as your parent or partner.
- Try not to overreport a *nyepa*, such as ***loong***.
- Complete the CSAT about who you *really* are, not the person you want to be.

MEDITATION ON A LOTUS FLOWER

Meditating on a beautiful lotus flower will help you to transform your mind and life. During this meditation, let go of negativity and, as a result, you will make healthier lifestyle choices. The internet has many photos of colorful lotus flowers.

To germinate, a lotus seed needs mud. The lotus seed turns mud into nourishment to sprout, rise, and bloom. Lotus flowers transform a swamp into a colorful garden.

Like a lotus, you can view "mud" in life as nourishment, not a threat. If so, you will transform challenges into opportunities for personal growth. Meditating on a lotus will strengthen you to do this ethical, spiritual work. You, too, will rise, bloom, and flourish.

Set up time to meditate each day. For example, visualize the lotus before getting out of bed in the morning and before going to sleep at night. See yourself as a lotus flower as you wash dishes. After parking your car, sit for a moment to contemplate the lotus. Take work breaks to reflect on the lotus. When you are angry, step back and imagine that you are a lotus.

How to Meditate on a Lotus Flower

- Sit comfortably in a straight-back chair, on a meditation cushion, or on the floor, or lie on your back with your arms comfortably stretched out by your side.
- Relax and straighten your back so that you can breathe deeply.
- Breathe in a circular manner, through your nostrils, from your abdomen, slowly, deeply, evenly, with your in-breath the same length as your out-breath, and no break in between.
- As you breathe in a circular manner, visualize a lotus flower; when your mind wanders, bring it back to the lotus. Rather than visualizing a lotus flower, you may find it helpful to look at real lotus or a photo of a lotus.
- Notice the color, size, and beauty of the lotus flower.
- Think about how a lotus seed requires mud to germinate, rise, and bloom.
- Visualize yourself transforming the "mud" in your life into nourishment so that you rise to your best self and bloom like a lotus.
- At the end of your meditation, take this visualization into your everyday life.

In summary, a qualified, experienced Tibetan medicine practitioner will teach you about your constitution and how to keep the current level of your *loong, tripa,* and *baekan* consistent with their percentages in your constitution. Using the CSAT and LGT together on a regular basis will help you to understand your constitution and who you *really* are. You will learn which lifestyle choices promote health and happiness, and which ones don't. Meditating on a lotus flower will empower you to transform your mind and your life.

The CSAT research findings and our experience teaching Tibetan medicine suggest that you will do more accurate CSAT assessments if you first study the basic teachings of Tibetan medicine, as explained in this book. You will understand your constitution better if you learn about energy, the source of existence. The next chapter goes into detail about the five elements, the five sources of energy from which everything arises. You will find out how to keep your **earth, water, fire, air,** and **space** in balance with your constitution.

· 3 ·

Understand the Source of Your Existence

$\mathcal{T}$ibetan medicine teaches that all phenomena are composed of energy. *Joong-wa-nya* is the Tibetan term for the five sources of energy from which everything arises. These five profound metaphors are **earth**, **water**, **fire**, **air**, and **space**. Ancient Tibetans used words from the natural world to explain the complex energy infusing all phenomena. All suffering and disease are due to the five sources of energy, loosely translated as the five elements. All remedies come from the five elements.

Sa, or **earth**, means cold, structure, and solidity. *Chu*, or **water**, is moisture and cohesion. *Mey*, or **fire**, refers to heat. *Loong*, or **air**, is movement. *Namkha*, or **space**, allows the other four elements to coexist and interact. The four elements of **earth**, **water**, **fire**, and **air** continuously interact with each other in **space**, the fifth element. Like all living beings, you were born with **earth**, **water**, **fire**, **air**, and **space**.

Health results from balance, whereas imbalance leads to disease. This chapter explains the five elements, how to recognize when they are in or out of balance, and ways to reverse imbalance. The chapter ends with Tonglen Meditation, a powerful practice to cultivate compassion. Compassion is crucial to understand and live in harmony with the five elements.

HEALTH IS BALANCE AND DIS-EASE IS IMBALANCE

Five Elements and Three Primary Energies

Earth, water, fire, air, and **space** are inherent in each of your cells. *Joong-wa-nya* is all around you. Each element produces different body constituents.

How the Five Elements Manifest in the Body

- **Earth** manifests as muscle tissues, bones, nose, and sense of smell.
- **Water** manifests as blood, body fluids, tongue, and sense of taste.
- **Fire** manifests as body temperature, complexion, eyes, and sight.
- **Air** manifests as respiration, skin, and sense of touch.
- **Space** manifests as body cavities, ears, and hearing.

Earth, water, fire, and **air** manifest in the form of the three primary energies. The **air** element produces *loong* (movement) energy. The **fire** element transforms into *tripa* (hot) energy. **Earth** and **water** elements combine to form *baekan* (cold) energy. Each of the three primary energies has divisions and subdivisions. *Nyepa*, meaning defect, is the Tibetan term for the three primary energies, as explained in chapters 1 and 4.

The five elements and three primary energies are vital for life. They work together to produce mental and physical health. Because they are in a constant state of flux, your balance is delicate and in continuous need of adjustment. Understanding the relationship among all these components will help you to create a harmonious life.

Your Unique Nature

You were born with a unique mixture of *joong-wa-nya*. Because the five elements comprise the three primary energies, you also were born with a unique combination of the *nyepa*. Your individual makeup of these components is called your true nature, your inborn constitutional nature or, simply, your constitution.

Your unique inborn combination of the five elements and three primary energies influences your character, perspective, personality, emotions, temperament, body type, strengths, weaknesses, diseases to which you are susceptible, and everything else about you. The five elements and *nyepa* are integral to your physical, mental, and spiritual experience. Therefore, understanding the very source of your existence is essential for a healthy, happy life.

Interaction of the Five Elements and Three Primary Energies

Each of the five elements has subtle qualities that affect the *nyepa*. **Earth** and **water** manifest in *baekan* energy. **Earth** is oily, heavy, blunt, smooth, stable, and sticky. These characteristics aggravate *baekan* and pacify *loong*. The **water** element is fluid, cool, heavy, blunt, oily, and flexible. The qualities aggravate *baekan* and pacify *tripa*.

The **fire** element manifests in *tripa* energy, which is hot, sharp, moist, coarse, light, oily, and mobile. These characteristics aggravate *tripa* and pacify *baekan*. The **air** element manifests in *loong*, which is light, mobile, cold, coarse, non-oily, and dry. These qualities aggravate *loong* and pacify *baekan*.

You are healthy if you develop a harmonious relationship between your inner and outer elements. Suffering and disease result when the five elements in and around you are not in sync. To recover, you need to reverse the imbalance, bring your five elements back into balance with your constitution, and create health.

Interconnectedness

Everything in every dimension is composed of interactions between the five sources of energy. All five elements were essential for you to be conceived. Your conception resulted from the five elements, your mother's ovum, your father's sperm, your consciousness, and your karmic seeds. When you die, the five elements will dissolve in this order: **earth, water, fire, air,** and **space**. One element disintegrates. The next element in order becomes more pronounced before it, too, breaks down.

First, **earth** dissolves. As you become dehydrated, your extremities loosen. You lose the sense of sight and feel like you are sinking underground. Second, **water** dissolves. Your body orifices become dry and your hearing diminishes. Third, **fire** dissolves. You lose your body heat, thereby hampering your digestive system. Your sense of smell declines, and you have trouble inhaling. Fourth, **air** dissolves. Life-sustaining *loong* moves to your heart. Your heart and breathing stop, and your tongue thickens. You lose your sense of taste and touch. Finally, **space** dissolves, and you are dead. For details, read chapter 9 and Tibetan Buddhist books on this topic.

Throughout life, your relationship to the five elements determines the quality of your experience. The five elements affect you profoundly on a deep, instinctive level. If deprived of an element, you yearn for it. On a long airplane flight, you can't wait to be back on **earth** again. You crave **water** in a desert. In sweltering **heat**, you seek **cold**. You gasp for **air** if you can't breathe. When feeling crowded, you long for **space**.

Joong-wa-nya may seem insufficient to account for all diversity. However, the five elements have subtle, multiple divisions that affect everything. Their interactions give rise to each person, animal, and plant in all realms and all dimensions. The five elements are integrally involved in the complexities and source of all that exists.

The five elements provide philosophic, fundamental metaphors for explaining energy that is essential for life. Each element ranges from subtle to gross. An excess or lack of an element manifests in physical, energetic, mental, and spiritual dimensions. These dimensions are interconnected and interactive, rather than separate entities.

When you understand *joong-wa-nya*, you come to realize that all phenomena are part of the energy field. Everything is interconnected like waves in an ocean. Waves rise and fall, but the sea remains. Waves cannot be separated from the ocean but are comprised of the ocean. Likewise, no phenomenon is a separate entity. Everything is affected by everything else and affects everything else.

Which Elements Dominate?

Each of the five elements contains the other four elements. They work with and against each other in diverse interactions. For example, **air** supports a **fire** to grow larger, but **air** also can extinguish the **fire**. Balance of the elements is dynamic and changes to a lesser and greater extent depending on the situation.

You have a unique combination all five elements in each of your cells. To recognize which of your elements is stronger or weaker, pay attention to your consistent characteristics and behaviors. Generally, do you tend to be earthy, fluid, hotheaded, airy, or spacey? Which element describes you best? Try to figure out what, if any, elements are in excess or are deficient. As you get to know yourself, you will recognize when your elements are in balance and out of balance.

Countless variables can cause your five elements to go out of balance. Examples are your thoughts, diet, behavior, emotions, relationships, work, environment, and lifestyle. Also, you can balance the five elements with your thoughts, diet, behavior, emotions, relationships, work, environment, and lifestyle. You intuitively know how to balance your five elements, even if you aren't mindful of your internal wisdom. Learning more about each element will help you to understand yourself and how to create a state of balance amid continuous change.[1]

EARTH: COLD, STABILITY, STRUCTURE

The **earth** element provides the foundation for mind and body. **Earth** is in every cell of the body. However, **earth** is most apparent in muscle tissues, bones, nose, and sense of smell.

Balanced *Earth* Element

When your **earth** element is in balance with your constitution, you feel stable, grounded, and confident. You have similar qualities to a bountiful land that produces fruit, grains, and vegetables. Like **earth**, you are moist and fertile, instead of dry, barren, and useless. You deal productively with life, rather than being set in your ways.

Solid, you aren't easily knocked off balance. Like a mountain, you withstand the storms of life. You keep your priorities in mind, even during challenging situations, and you don't lose touch with what is important. Impulsivity doesn't easily sweep aside your intentions. You are consistent, responsible, and independent. If you evolve to a higher spiritual level, compassion and wisdom ground you, and you are aware of your luminous, ultimate mind.

*Increased **Earth** Element*

If your **earth** element rises too high, you become dull, slow, and lethargic. Your thinking lacks inspiration and creativity. Too solid, you get stuck and are unable to bring about change. Your problems seem insurmountable, and you personally identify with them. You may become depressed and resigned to unacceptable situations.

The lazier you become, the more you procrastinate and don't get things done. You sleep too much, but after you wake up, you still feel tired. Either you withdraw and don't talk, or, if you start talking, you can't seem to stop. When you try to meditate, you fall asleep. You habitually are late for appointments, or you are punctual to the minute. Because you lack heat, you become cold and set in your ways.

If your **earth** element is too high, you can decrease it by eating spicy, warm, and light foods, such as seasoned, lightly cooked vegetables. Exercise vigorously and regularly to raise your metabolism and heat. Expand your thinking. See things from diverse perspectives. Avoid sleeping during the day. Lighten your life, body, and thinking.

*Decreased **Earth** Element*

When your **earth** element falls too low, you feel ungrounded and dissatisfied. You have trouble sleeping through the night. Unfocused, you can't complete what you begin. Without an anchor, you become flighty and anxious, and you don't feel at home at any place. You keep looking for what will ground you and make you feel secure.

If your **earth** element is insufficient, you can balance it by becoming grounded. Stay home. Be quiet. Work in your garden or walk in nature. Train your mind to focus. Eat heavier foods such as potatoes and other root vegetables. Avoid caffeine and similar stimulants. Practice steadiness of mind and body. Stability will help you to meditate and develop wisdom. Create a safe home, healthy relationships, and satisfying work.

WATER: MOISTURE AND COHESION

The **water** element is in every cell of your body. However, **water** is most prevalent in your blood, body fluids, tongue, and sense of taste.

Balanced **Water** Element

When your **water** element is in balance, you feel comfortable with your life. You are fluid and flexible. Rather than being rigid, you easily maneuver through the various challenges in your life. You change what you can change and accept everything else. Because you are comfortable with impermanence, you feel peaceful amid continuous change. You enjoy your relationships, work, situations, and everything else in your life. Grateful for your precious human life, you reach out to help others. You are not affected adversely by situations around you. Gratefulness wells up inside you.

Increased **Water** Element

If your **water** element is excessive, you have difficulty controlling your emotions. You are tearful, tossed around, and immersed in self-pity. Hypersensitive, you react emotionally to whatever occurs. You avoid what is difficult, even if you must give up your important goals. Unable to think clearly, you let your responsibilities slide. You float through life and stay with what you should change.

When your **water** element rises too high, you need to reduce it. Develop equanimity, rather than react emotionally to whatever occurs. Heal self-pity by practicing self-compassion, compassion toward yourself. Treat yourself gently as you do a baby. Behave with compassion toward everyone and everything. Fulfill your responsibilities and make changes as needed.

Decreased **Water** Element

Insufficient **water** element results in an arid, infertile life lacking in flexibility, joy, and gratitude. You are uncomfortable with yourself and other people. Because you are looking for happiness outside yourself, you try to do more and accumulate more. You believe that life will be better if only you develop a new relationship, or you get a different job, more money and honors, new clothes, or whatever else you desire. When you try to meditate, you engage in dualistic thinking, rather than seeing the interconnectedness of everything.

If your **water** element is deficient, you can bring it into balance by recognizing your suffering. Create a life that comforts you and gives you joy. Set realistic goals. Change what you can change and learn to accept peacefully what you can't change.

FIRE: HEAT

Like the other four elements, the **fire** element is in each cell of your body. **Fire** is most apparent in your body temperature, complexion, eyes, and sight.

Balanced *Fire* Element

When your **fire** element is in balance, you initiate projects and accomplish goals. **Fire** nurtures you instead of destroying you. Because your digestive heat is strong, you digest food properly and burn off toxins. Your face shines with energy, and your body temperature is normal. Rather than being hostile and angry, you transform heat into compassion. You are intuitive and enthusiastic. **Fire** helps you to expand your consciousness, think clearly, and make healthy choices. You set goals and meet them. A wise leader, you bring people together to benefit the community.

Increased *Fire* Element

If you have too much **fire** element, you become reactive and agitated. You lash out angrily, without thinking, even when you drive in traffic and need to focus on safety. Lacking patience and tolerance, you are annoyed by anyone who disagrees with you or is different from you. You easily feel irritated and run over other people to get what you want. Rather than wait for someone else to speak, you interrupt, dominate the conversation, and finish the person's sentences. Over time, you develop inflammations, infections, skin rashes, and even hair loss as your body tries to reduce its heat.

When your **fire** is elevated, you move too fast and try to do too much. You can't sit still because you always have something more to do. Silence and stillness bore you. If you try to meditate, your monkey mind won't slow down.

Notice if your **fire** is too high and then decrease it. When you are angry, take time out to cool down. Better yet, root out anger and practice self-compassion. Cultivate compassion for others by asking, "How can I help?"

To cool your **fire**, avoid spicy foods, vigorous exercise, alcohol, and "hot" situations. Eat cooling foods, such as potatoes and asparagus. Engage in cooling actions like listening to peaceful music, doing gentle yoga poses, and walking quietly in nature.

Decreased *Fire Element*

When your **fire** falls too low, you lack vitality, inspiration, and enthusiasm. You don't enjoy your work, your relationships, or anything else. Intellectually, you are quick, but you don't apply what you learn and accomplish your goals. If your **fire** is disturbed, you are susceptible to developing digestive, endocrine, and/or metabolic problems.

If your **fire** element is insufficient, you can increase it by warming up. Do the opposite of what you need to do to decrease your **fire** element. Bring your **fire** into balance by creating a happy life. Do worthwhile work and accomplish your goals.

AIR: MOVEMENT

The **air** element, like the other elements, is in every cell of your body. **Air** is most apparent in your respiration, skin, and sense of touch. Of all the five elements, **air** is *the* essential element for life. All five elements are necessary. Without **air**, however, you will die quickly.

The **air** element pervades everyone and everything. **Air** is involved with every movement of your mind and body. When your body moves, your thoughts move, and vice versa. For example, you can't sit still if your thoughts jump around like a monkey. **Air** is related to supreme vitality, the most refined, subtle part of the body. Supreme vitality resides primarily in the heart center, but the effects spread throughout the body.

Balanced Air Element

When **air** is in balance, you are flexible in mind and body. You see what's positive in challenging situations and you develop understanding. If things go wrong, you are grateful for what goes right. You create, change, and communicate because of **air**. Balanced **air** allows you to be curious and see things from various perspectives. **Air** connects all phenomena. During meditation, **air** helps to expand your consciousness.

Increased Air Element

If you have too much **air** element, **earth** and **water** may be deficient. You lack stability and contentment and have difficulty focusing. When you are in one place, another location looks better. You go to the new one, and you want to be somewhere else. Because you are dis-satisfied (lack of satisfaction), you don't find comfort in the way things are.

When even a small challenge arises, you quickly become frustrated. You ruminate instead of solving the problem. Your confidence crumbles, and you can't sleep. You are anxious and flighty. Before you express one thought, another thought rises in your mind. Thoughts race through your head, and you don't know what to do with them. You talk quickly and jump from one topic to another one. Ungrounded, you are like the wind that blows this way and that way.

If your **air** is too high, you can reestablish balance by calming your mind and body. Slow down. Avoid stimulants such as coffee. Become grounded by going home, being silent, and taking a nap. Do gentle yoga poses. Meditate. Walk safely in nature. Listen to beautiful, calming music. Get a massage or Reiki treatment. Select earthy friends, not individuals who are "airy." Set up a regular lifestyle. Eat meals and engage in activities that keep you warm.

Decreased Air Element

If you lead an anxious, stressful life, your **air** initially increases to support your choices. Eventually, you deplete your **air**. As in making tea, boiling water too long produces steam, and then you don't have enough water left for tea. Without enough **air**, you can't breathe deeply. Life suffocates you. You feel stuck, but you lack energy to make needed changes. When meditating, you can't focus, and you fall asleep.

If your **air** is disturbed, you become impatient. You can't concentrate and sit still. Questions keep coming to mind. You feel like you must find answers right away, but you don't know which way to turn. Your mind is in constant turmoil.

Anxiety causes **air** to go out of balance and results from **air** being out of balance. You complain that aches and pains move around your body and come and go. Worried about the past, you are apprehensive about the future. Rather than resolve your problems, you compulsively focus on the causes and symptoms. You become prone to developing a chronic, wasting illness.

Whether your **air** is too high, too low, and/or disturbed, you need to figure out why you are anxious and resolve the issues. Change what you can change and accept everything else. Eat food to ground you, such as potatoes and other root vegetables that grow underground. Take steps to sleep well. When your **air** is in balance, your anxiety will decrease. Then you will be able to focus and accomplish your goals.

SPACE: ALLOWS THE OTHER ELEMENTS TO INTERACT

The **space** element, like the other four elements, is in every cell of your body. Everything arises from **space**, exists in **space**, and dissolves into **space**. Even so, **space** is most evident in your body cavities, ears, and hearing.

Balanced *Space* Element

When your **space** element is balanced, you have enough time, emotional capacity, and tolerance. You can accommodate whatever arises. Everything fits, without too much or too little. You don't dissociate from your experiences or become immersed in them. Your life, work, and home have enough **space** for everything.

You aren't caught up in everything that arises because you feel free. Rather be tossed around, you behave with equanimity. You live up to your most important values. Instead of blaming other people for your problems, you take responsibility to create a harmonious life. You see challenges realistically and deal well with them.

Increased *Space* Element

When you have too much **space** or **space** dominates your other four elements, you are "spacey" and have difficulty connecting with other people. You develop superficial views. Rootless, you drift through life. You don't feel like life has meaning. When you try to meditate, you easily get distracted. Lacking awareness, you feel lost and out of touch. Because you can't focus, you aren't able to accomplish your goals. You lose interest in your family, career, home, and everything else.

To reestablish balance in your **space** element, create a meaningful life. Cultivate loving relationships and do worthwhile, enjoyable work. Create comfortable, clean home and work environments. Engage in acts of loving-kindness. Train your mind to focus. Counteract being spacey. Accept who you are and be a positive influence for others.

Decreased *Space* Element

Too little **space** allows the other four elements to dominate your life. You become obsessed with whatever occurs, no matter how big or small, and you feel out of control. Everything seems insurmountable. "Stuff" that fills your thoughts and life paralyzes you. Rather than set priorities, you never have enough time for what you want to do. You feel frustrated by yourself, family, work, home, and everything else.

When you have too little **space**, it's time to clean out your mind, body, home, work, and life. Learn to say no. Slow down your life. Spend more time at home and in nature. Resolve your difficulties. Forgive and let go of resentments. Free yourself of entanglements.

TONGLEN MEDITATION

In the Tibetan language, Tonglen literally means "giving and taking." Tonglen Meditation is a well-known Tibetan Buddhist practice for cultivating compassion for yourself and other people. Doing Tonglen can bring the five elements into balance and keep them in balance. Beginners to advanced meditators can benefit from Tonglen. By practicing Tonglen regularly, you open your heart, heal your mind, and transform your life.

Because of karma, negative thinking gives rise to unhealthy lifestyle choices that result in harmful consequences. The three mental poisons depress the immune system and close the heart center. Negativity produces imbalance, suffering, and disease.

Tonglen will help you to deal effectively with challenging people and situations. If you let yourself get angry and frustrated at someone, you are likely to make things worse. Instead do Tonglen for the individual. You will transform your mental poisons into compassion and enhance your immune system. Tonglen may not change someone else, but it will change you and your relationship to the person.

How to Do Tonglen Meditation: Breathe in Suffering and Breathe Out Compassion

- **Sit or lie down comfortably with a straight back**: Relax your body, turn inside, halfway or fully close your eyes, and focus on your breath.
- **Engage in circular breathing**: Breathe slowly, deeply, and evenly through your nostrils, from your abdomen, with the in-breath the same length as the out-breath, and no break between the in-breath and out-breath.
- **Do Tonglen for yourself**: As you breathe in, let your greed, attachment, anger, jealousy, delusion, fear, confusion, sadness, and other negativity come to the surface. Breathe out this negativity and fill yourself with compassion.
- **Do Tonglen for someone you love**: Breathe in your loved one's suffering, like black smoke, into your heart center, and breathe out compassion to the person. Your loved one wants to be happy, but too often makes poor choices that produce suffering instead. Open your heart to your loved one.
- **Do Tonglen for someone, such as a store clerk, about whom you feel neutral**: Breathe in the person's suffering, like black smoke, into your heart center, and breathe out compassion to the person. Like everyone else, this individual wants to be happy

but may make the mistake of producing suffering instead. Open your heart to the person.

- **Do Tonglen for someone you don't like**: Breathe in the person's suffering, like black smoke, into your heart center, and breathe out compassion to the individual. This challenging individual wants to be happy but is suffering because of mental poisons. Open your heart to the person.
- **Do Tonglen for the world**: Breathe in the world's suffering, like black smoke, into your heart center, and breathe out compassion to the world. Open your heart to the world's suffering.
- **Purify yourself**: At the end of your meditation, visualize the suffering you breathed in as black smoke in your heart center. Breathe out this black smoke completely, or this negativity could cause suffering for you. Then fill your heart and your whole being with compassion toward yourself, all living beings, and the world.

In summary, **earth, water, fire, air**, and **space** provide an explanation for the complex energy that infuses everyone and everything. By learning about the five sources of your existence, you come to recognize when they are in balance and out of balance. However, understanding the five elements is not sufficient for healing and happiness. You will benefit by finding out more about your three primary energies.

The next chapter explains *loong, tripa*, and *baekan*. You will learn to recognize their ebb and flow, when they are in balance, and when they are out of balance. Keeping your *nyepa* consistent with your inborn constitution is essential for your health and happiness.

· 4 ·

Keep Your Three Primary Energies in Balance

$\mathcal{T}$ibetan medicine teaches that all phenomena are composed of *joong-wa-nya*. This Tibetan word means the five sources of energy from which all phenomena arise. These five energy sources, loosely translated as five elements, describe the complex energy that infuses everyone and everything. To name these metaphors, ancient Tibetans used terms from nature: **earth**, **water**, **fire**, **air**, and **space**.

The five elements interact to form three principal energies: *loong*, *tripa*, and *baekan*. *Loong*, movement energy, is based on the **air** element. *Tripa*, hot energy, arises from the **fire** element. *Baekan*, cold energy, combines the **water** element and the **earth** element. Each of the three primary energies has divisions and subdivisions that interact continuously. All three primary energies are essential for life.

Like all living beings, you were born with a unique combination of *loong*, *tripa*, and *baekan*. Your combination of the three primary energies is called your true nature, your inborn constitution or, simply, your constitution. In Western terms, your constitution is like your genes and DNA. To create health and happiness, you need to make lifestyle choices that support your unique constitution.

Nyepa is the Tibetan term for *loong*, *tripa*, and *baekan*. *Nyepa* means defect or fault. If in a state of imbalance, the three principal energies become seeds of suffering and disease. When in balance, they work together to produce mental and physical health. Your *nyepa* are in balance when their current percentages are about the same as their percentages in your inborn constitution.

Developing understanding of your three primary energies will help you to keep them in sync with your constitution. This chapter explains why *loong, tripa,* and *baekan* can become defects, analyzes each of them, and describes how they work together to promote health. The chapter ends with Alternate Nostril Breathing, a meditation that promotes balance in the *nyepa*.

NYEPA: DEFECT

Channels and Chakras

Loong, tripa, and *baekan* flow in an interconnected network of energy channels or meridians. According to some estimates, the body has at least seventy-two thousand energy channels. This complex network connects the external and internal parts of the body. Like the three primary energies, the energy channels are essential for life.

Loong energy flows in twenty-four thousand channels. The primary *loong* channel in the center of the body is called *uma* in Tibetan and *shushumna* in Sanskrit. This channel runs inside the spinal column from the base of the spine to the crown of the head.

Tripa energy flows in twenty-four thousand channels that carry solar, active, hot, light energy. The primary *tripa* channel is to the right of the *loong* channel, running along the spinal cord from the base of the spine to the crown of the head. In Tibetan, this channel is called *roma*; the Sanskrit term is *pingala*. This hot energy channel is connected to the right nostril, left brain, and sympathetic nervous system.

Baekan energy flows in twenty-four thousand channels that carry lunar, passive, cold, heavy energy. The main *baekan* channel is on the left side of the body, running along the spinal cord from the base of the spine to the crown of the head. The Tibetan name for this *baekan* channel is *kyangma*; the Sanskrit term is *ida*. This cold energy channel is connected to the left nostril, right brain, and parasympathetic nervous system.

The channels intersect at energy centers called chakras. The body has seven main chakras from the base of the spine to the crown of the head. They are named Base Chakra, Sacral Chakra, Solar Plexus Chakra, Heart Chakra, Throat Chakra, Brow Chakra or Third Eye, and Crown Chakra. Consciousness resides in each of these energy centers but primarily in the Heart Chakra.

Imbalance on Distant and Immediate Levels

Disease is caused by imbalance on the distant level and immediate level. On the distant level, the cause of disequilibrium and disease is ignorance about the true nature of the self. Tibetan medicine, influenced strongly by Tibetan Buddhist philosophy, teaches that an intrinsic self doesn't exist. You do not have an independent self. Ignorance, called *ma-rig-pa* in Tibetan, is the general distant cause of all disorders. Fundamental ignorance of the self produces self-grasping and a focus on "I."

Narcissism is the seed of the three mental poisons, called *dug-gsum* in Tibetan. The three mental poisons are: (1) greed, attachment, and desire; (2) anger, hostility, and aggression; and (3) delusion, confusion, and closed-mindedness. When you engage in this negativity, you are likely to make unhealthy lifestyle choices that cause you to become extremely vulnerable. The three mental poisons are the specific distant cause of disequilibrium and disease.

Loong*, *tripa*, and *baekan are the immediate cause of imbalance and dysfunction. When in balance, the *nyepa* support health and happiness. However, they manifest as characteristics of disease when out of balance. Your state of balance and health become disrupted when you choose to expose yourself to these conditions: unwholesome diet, improper behavior, adverse seasonal changes, and other negative factors.

To be happy and healthy, you need to make choices that keep the current levels of your ***loong*, *tripa*, and *baekan*** consistent with their levels in your constitution. Unhealthy choices produce imbalance in your *nyepa*. Rather than sustain you, they become defects.

A primary energy is out of balance if it rises too high, falls too low, or becomes disturbed. Ordinarily, ***loong*** goes out of balance first. You are anxious and can't sleep. Thoughts race through your mind. You make poor choices about what to eat and drink and don't digest your food well. Toxins accumulate. If one primary energy becomes unbalanced, the other two primary energies are likely to go out of balance, too. Over time, this imbalanced state of the *nyepa* can lead to complicated illnesses such as cancer.

Because everything is composed of energy, all phenomena, including your body, are impermanent. Attachment to what is in flux produces mental disturbance. For example, you may try to make a relationship permanent, even though you and the other person are constantly changing. This approach isn't realistic or beneficial.

These teachings highlight the dynamic relationship between mind, body, and environment. Positivity and negativity affect you on every level down to your *nyepa* and the five elements, the very source of your existence. In a nutshell, you can't free yourself of suffering and disease without rooting out the causes of the three mental poisons.

Three Primary Energies and Three Mental Poisons

Engaging in the three mental poisons has a devastating effect on your *nyepa*. Greed, attachment, and desire cause and result from *loong* imbalance. Anger, hostility, and aggression cause and result from *tripa* imbalance. Delusion, confusion, and closed-mindedness cause and result from *baekan* imbalance. The three mental poisons disrupt the dynamic equilibrium of your three primary energies that are essential for life. If *loong*, *tripa*, and *baekan* go out of balance and become defects, they transform into seeds of disease.

Positive thoughts help you to make healthy lifestyle choices. Behaving with compassion enhances your immune system and causes your mind and body to function smoothly. You keep your three primary energies in sync with your constitution. Your *loong*, *tripa*, and *baekan* maintain their functions on mental and physical levels. In a balanced state, your *nyepa* help you to live a happy, healthy life.

The *nyepa* cause harm if you engage in the three mental poisons. Even fifteen minutes of anger increases blood pressure, heart rate, and breathing rate, and depresses the immune system. Over time, these physiological changes have disastrous effects. The energy channels and chakras become blocked, and energy no longer flows freely through them. The mind and body deteriorate.

You can free yourself from the three mental poisons by recognizing that you don't have a separate, intrinsic self. Coming to understand emptiness and interdependence is an antidote to ignorance. Nothing in the universe at macro and micro levels exists by itself. Everything is interconnected and depends on everything else. For example, your existence depends on innumerable variables such as your parents, genes, consciousness, karma, behavior, diet, environment, socialization, associates, and work. You are **empty** of an independent self.

To balance your *loong*, *tripa*, and *baekan*, you need to heal the three mental poisons and develop harmony within yourself, as well as with everyone and everything. Develop understanding about the inter-dependent nature of the self. Training your mind transforms the three mental poisons into positive behavior. This process decreases the faults and enhances the strengths of your constitution. Learning more about your *nyepa*, as well as factors that maintain their balance, will help you to do this ethical, spiritual work.

LOONG: MOVEMENT ENERGY

*Functions and Subdivisions of **Loong***

Loong energy, translated loosely as wind, resides primarily in the genitals, large intestine, and lower part of the body. *Loong* regulates all movement, both physical movement and thoughts in the mind. When the body is moving, thoughts are moving, and vice versa.

Loong controls blood circulation, digestion, menstruation, urination, defecation, and development and delivery of the fetus. Because of *loong*, you can breathe, your heart pumps blood, your lymph circulates through your body, and you can swallow food and beverages. You can spit, cough, burp, sneeze, and talk.

Loong serves as an essential conduit between mind and body. Balanced *loong* promotes creativity and sustains the internal organs, sense organs, and entire body. Like wind, though, *loong* quickly can vary from cold to hot, and vice versa. If your *loong* is out of balance, your mind and body can feel cold one minute and hot a few minutes later, and then back to cold again.

Loong has five subdivisions. They are life-sustaining *loong*, ascending *loong*, pervasive *loong*, fire-accompanying *loong*, and descending *loong*. These subdivisions reside in particular sites of the body. Each subdivision has specific functions.

Life-sustaining *loong (sok-zin-loong)* resides in the Crown Chakra. This *loong* is similar to *prana*, or life force in Ayurveda, and *chi* in Chinese medicine. Life-sustaining *loong* moves through the throat and chest regions. It supports consciousness and is the source of the other subdivisions of *loong*.

Ascending *loong (gyen-gyu-loong)* resides in the Throat Chakra and chest, and moves through the nose, tongue, and larynx. Its functions are to produce the voice and speech, clear the sensory organs, and sharpen the memory. Ascending *loong* gives the body physical strength and creates the glow of a good complexion. It provides willpower and diligence to accomplish tasks.

Pervasive *loong (kyab-chay)* resides in the Heart Chakra but pervades the whole body. This *loong* promotes blood circulation and the lymphatic system. It regulates mental and physical movement, such as stretching, bending, walking. Pervasive *loong* opens and closes the body orifices.

Fire-accompanying *loong (mey-nyam)* resides in the Navel Chakra and stomach and moves through the gastrointestinal tract. This *loong* accompanies *tripa* digestive heat. Fire-accompanying *loong* helps to digest food, separate nutrients from waste products, and move the bowels. It aids in maturing the bodily constituents.

Descending *loong (thoor-sel)* resides in the Genital Chakra and rectum. This *loong* moves through the large intestine, urinary bladder, thighs, and genitals. It promotes expulsion of semen, urine, feces, menstruation, and child delivery.

Characteristics of **Loong**

Loong has six distinct characteristics. These qualities distinguish *loong* from *tripa* and *baekan*. Because everyone has *loong* energy, each person exhibits these characteristics to some degree. These qualities are most evident if *loong* dominates your constitution.

Six Characteristics of **Loong** Energy

1. **Rough**: *Loong* regulates blood flow; the quality of blood is rough. A *loong* person has a rough tongue and skin and considers any discomfort to be unbearable.
2. **Light**: *Loong* diseases respond lightly or easily to treatment. A *loong* individual experiences a light sensation in mind and body.
3. **Cold**: A *loong* person typically feels cold and desires warm food and environment.
4. **Subtle**: *Loong* easily enters any location of the body.
5. **Hard**: *Loong* growths do not form pus easily. A *loong* person tends to have hard bowel movements and be constipated. *Loong* fevers ordinarily do not mature.

6. **Mobile**: A *loong* individual may suffer from delirium, halluci-
   nations, and hysteria. *Loong* pulse, swellings, growths, and pain
   fluctuate and change.

Prevalence of *Loong*

The three *nyepa* continuously rise and fall during each twenty-four-
hour period. *Loong* energy is highest from about 3 a.m. to 7 a.m. and
about 3 p.m. to 7 p.m. *Tripa* energy is highest from about 11 a.m. to 3
p.m. and about 11 p.m. to 3 a.m. *Baekan* energy is highest from about
7 a.m. to 11 a.m. and about 7 p.m. to 11 p.m.

If you are asleep during the early morning *loong* period, you may
experience wisdom dreams that provide insight about life. The morning *loong* period is an ideal time to meditate. Don't stay in bed until the
morning *baekan* period begins, or you may be tired all day long. Work,
exercise, and eat lightly during the afternoon *loong* period.

Imbalance of *Loong*

Loong results from and causes the mental poison of greed, attachment,
and desire. When you engage in this negativity, you feel dissatisfied
with life. You want things to be different from what they are. This dis-
satisfaction causes *loong* to go out of balance and produces stress-related
problems. If *loong* dominates your constitution, a *loong* imbalance is
more serious than if *tripa* and/or *baekan* are dominant.

When your *loong* is out of balance, you experience insomnia,
nervousness, anxiety, mood swings, depression, heart palpitations, indigestion, swirling thoughts, emotional distance, headaches, anxiety, and
depression. Chronic *loong* imbalance can result in mental illness and/or
addiction to alcohol, drugs, relationships, food, sex, work, success, possessions, gambling, emotions, religion, ideas, or anything else.

How to Balance *Loong*

Meditate on impermanence to heal greed, attachment, and desire.
Come to accept that everything continuously changes. Rather than
allow thoughts to race in your head, train your mind to focus. Reduce

stress, become grounded, and do what is calming. Cultivate mindfulness and joy in the moment.

You can calm your mind and body by going home and being quiet. Rather than talk, listen to pleasant music. Take a nap if you are tired. Walk in nature. Spend time with family and friends you enjoy. Avoid angry, hostile people. Do meaningful work. Live, work, and sleep peacefully. Create a happy, healthy life.

You can bring *loong* into balance by what you eat and drink. Eat calming, moisturizing, warm, easily digested food. Examples are rice, warm soups, bananas, and slightly cooked vegetables. Boil water and cool it enough to drink. Avoid caffeine and other stimulants.

If you have a *loong* constitution, you will benefit from dairy products, if you can digest them. Eat mild spices and warm, protein-rich foods. Choose sweet, sour, and salty tastes. Avoid bitter foods, such as raw fruits and vegetables, and salads with acidic vegetables such as tomatoes. To keep your digestive heat high, stay away from cold foods and beverages, such as cold salads and iced drinks.

With a *loong* constitution, you will thrive in a beautiful, peaceful, healthy environment. Keep your home well heated and well ventilated. Wear clothing that helps you to stay warm. Respond promptly to the needs of your mind and body.

TRIPA: HOT ENERGY

Functions and Subdivisions of *Tripa*

Tripa energy, loosely translated as bile, resides in the body's midsection, particularly in the liver and gall bladder. The function of *tripa* is to regulate heat in the mind and body. *Tripa* is responsible for hunger, thirst, metabolism, growth, development, digestion, a radiant complexion, and absorption of food and ideas. This hot energy promotes clear thinking, courage, determination, intelligence, and achievement of goals.

Like *loong*, *tripa* has five subdivisions. *Tripa* subdivisions are digestive *tripa*, color-transforming *tripa*, accomplishing *tripa*, sight *tripa*, and complexion-clearing *tripa*. They reside in specific sites of the body and have particular functions.

Digestive *tripa (jhu-chay)* is located between the stomach and intestines, between the sites of undigested food and digested food. This *tripa* generates body heat. It digests food and beverages and separates nutrients from waste. Digestive *tripa* assists the other four types of *tripa* to function well.

Color-transforming *tripa (daang-gyur)*, which resides in the liver, provides the color of all body constituents including red blood and white bones. Accomplishing *tripa (dhup-chay)* in the heart promotes courage, pride, and intelligence, and assists in accomplishing goals. Sight *tripa (thong-chay)* in the eyes enables sight. Complexion-clearing *tripa (dhok-sel)* in the skin is responsible for a healthy and lustrous complexion.

Characteristics of **Tripa**

Tripa energy has seven distinct characteristics. These qualities distinguish *tripa* from *loong* and *baekan*. Everyone exhibits these characteristics to some degree because each person has *tripa* energy. These characteristics are more pronounced if *tripa* dominates your constitution.

Seven Characteristics of **Tripa** Energy

1. **Oily**: A *tripa* person has slight oiliness of complexion and skin.
2. **Sharp**: A *tripa* individual is quick to act. *Tripa* diseases occur suddenly, fevers mature quickly, and swellings easily form and give off pus.
3. **Hot**: *Tripa* heats the body, causes thirst, and increases body temperature. A *tripa* person desires cool foods and beverages and seeks a cool environment.
4. **Light**: A *tripa* individual responds to treatment lightly or readily.
5. **Foul-smelling**: A *tripa* person has foul-smelling sweat, breath, urine, and feces.
6. **Purgative**: A *tripa* individual tends to have loose bowel movements.
7. **Moist or liquid**: A *tripa* person's phlegm and blood have a moist, liquid quality.

Prevalence of **Tripa**

This hot energy is highest from about 11 a.m. to 3 p.m. and 11 p.m. to 3 a.m. During the daytime *tripa* period, eat your biggest meal. Your digestive fire is at the highest level then, and you are more likely to digest food properly. Also, during this period do your work, without getting too warmed up. If the weather is hot, you may need to stay quiet right after your noon meal so that you don't get overheated.

Go to bed no later than 10:30 p.m. Sleep soundly during the night *tripa* period. Then *tripa* can burn off toxins in your mind and body. You will awake feeling refreshed. If you don't sleep deeply at this time, toxins can accumulate and cause disease.

Imbalance of **Tripa**

Engaging in the mental poison of anger, hostility, and aggression increases *tripa*. This hot energy promotes rage, violence, trying to do too much, and leading a hectic life. Elevated *tripa* destroys bodily constituents such as blood and muscle. High *tripa* can produce hair loss as the body tries to decrease heat.

Too much *tripa* produces hot disorders and a feeling of being "hot under the collar." Examples of hot disorders are elevated temperature, rashes, itchy skin, metabolic and endocrine problems, liver dysfunction, and indigestion. Elevated *tripa* can cause inflammations, infections, and rapid pulse. Menopausal women may experience hot flashes and night sweats. If *tripa* rules your constitution, *tripa* imbalance is more serious than if *loong* and/or *baekan* are dominant.

How to Balance **Tripa**

To heal anger, hostility, and aggression, meditate on and develop self-compassion. Furthermore, practice compassion toward everyone. Compassion enhances the immune system, opens the heart, and promotes harmony. Rather than a feeling, compassion is a philosophical stance, a yearning for all beings to be free of suffering and the causes of suffering.

Treat all people with kindness, no matter how they behave. Each person is of your own kind, not a different species. Clear thinking that is not corrupted by anger will help you to set appropriate limits if someone mistreats you.

If *tripa* rises too high, do what is cooling. Slow down. Take a break. Sit quietly. Meditate on your breath. Walk safely in nature. Listen to music that cools you down. Do gentle yoga postures and breathing. Fill your mind with cooling thoughts.

To cool *tripa*, avoid foods and beverages that heat you up, such as fish, chicken, red meat, spices, ginger, alcohol, and caffeine. Instead, drink cooling beverages such as boiled, cooled pure water. Eat cooling foods, such as potatoes, beets, carrots, and other root vegetables. Root vegetables are cooling because they grow in the earth away from the sun. In general, fresh greens and cold salads cool *tripa*.

If you have a *tripa* constitution, you are likely to thrive in a cool environment and climate. Wear clothes that decrease your body heat. Do cooling work that you enjoy. Focus on one activity at a time and avoid multitasking. Exercise in a manner that doesn't cause you to sweat and become overheated. Steer clear of sunbathing, saunas, jogging, hot yoga, and other heat-producing activities. Create a peaceful, cool lifestyle.

BAEKAN: COLD ENERGY

Functions and Subdivisions of **Baekan**

Baekan energy, loosely translated as phlegm, resides in the head and upper part of the body. When out of balance, *baekan* descends to the lower part of the body. The function of *baekan* is to maintain stability of the mind, as well as the structure, firmness, and smoothness of the body. **Baekan** generates patience and compassion. This cold energy lubricates joints, induces sleep, and regulates lymphatic function.

Like *loong* and *tripa*, *baekan* has five subdivisions. The *baekan* subdivisions are supporting *baekan*, decomposing *baekan*, experiencing *baekan*, satisfying *baekan*, and connecting *baekan*. They reside in specific sites of the body and have particular functions.

Supporting *baekan (then-chay)* resides in the chest region, particularly around the upper ribs and breastbone. It supports the other types of *baekan* by providing moisture and structure. Decomposing *baekan* *(nyak-chay)* is in the site of undigested food (stomach). This *baekan* breaks down food into a semiliquid paste in preparation for the next digestive stage.

Experiencing *baekan (nyong-chay)* resides on the tongue where it detects the taste and textures of food. Satisfying *baekan (tseem-chay)*, in the head and neck, facilitates the sensory organs to function. Connecting *baekan (jor-chay)*, located in all the joints, lubricates the joints so that the body can stretch, retract, and bend.

Characteristics of Baekan

Baekan energy has seven distinct characteristics. These qualities distinguish *baekan* from *loong* and *tripa*. Everyone has *baekan* energy and exhibits these characteristics to some degree. These characteristics are obvious if *baekan* dominates your constitution.

Seven Characteristics of Baekan Energy

1. **Oily**: A *baekan* person's diarrhea, vomiting, feces, and blood have an oily quality.
2. **Cool**: A *baekan* individual generally lacks physical warmth, especially when ill, and seeks warm food, beverages, and environments.
3. **Heavy**: A *baekan* person feels a heaviness or lethargy in mind and body and responds slowly to treatment.
4. **Blunt**: A *baekan* individual's joints are round because flesh covers them.
5. **Smooth**: A *baekan* person's tongue, skin, and blood have a soft quality. Symptoms of a *baekan* disease are soft. A *baekan* person feels little pain.
6. **Stable**: A *baekan* individual's swellings, growths, and pain don't fluctuate much, and bowel movements tend to be medium, rather than hard or loose.
7. **Sticky**: A *baekan* person's vomit, feces, blood, phlegm, and saliva are sticky.

Prevalence of Baekan

Baekan energy is highest from about 7 a.m. to 11 a.m. and about 7 p.m. to 11 p.m. You are best off getting out of bed during the morning *loong* period. Increase your metabolism and heat by doing gentle exercises and eating a nutritious, warm breakfast. As your *baekan* energy rises, you will feel grounded and able to focus on work. You are likely to feel sluggish and cold if you get up during the morning *baekan* period. Unless you generate heat, you may procrastinate and have difficulty accomplishing your goals for the day.

During the evening *baekan* period, prepare to sleep by slowing your thinking and body. Take a leisurely walk. Spend time with enjoyable family and friends. Read a relaxing book. Listen to calming music. Go to bed and turn out the lights before the evening *baekan* period ends so that you sleep soundly during the night *tripa* period.

Imbalance of **Baekan**

Delusion, confusion, and closed-mindedness cause and result from *baekan* energy. *Baekan* imbalance produces cold behavior because of insufficient heat and too much solidity. Examples of cold behaviors are procrastination, lethargy, sleepiness, and inertia.

Too much *baekan* promotes accumulation of fatty tissue and obesity. A *baekan* person is vulnerable to developing diabetes, sinus congestion, asthma, colds, edema, and kidney dysfunction. If *baekan* dominates your constitution, a *baekan* imbalance is more serious for you than if you have a *loong* and/or *tripa* constitution. *Baekan* energy is heavy and viscous. When *baekan* manifests in the brain, it can obscure intelligence and clarity and cause confusion. Dementia may result in part from a long-term imbalance in *baekan*.

How to Balance **Baekan**

Meditate on and develop wisdom to heal confusion, delusion, and closed-mindedness. Wake up! Take off the blinders and see things as they *really* are, not the way you want them to be. Expand your thinking to understand other people's perspectives. Create an enlightened mind.

If your *baekan* energy is too high, think and do what will decrease your cold and heat you up. Engage in activities that are warm and dry. Exercise vigorously and often to increase your metabolism and take off pounds. Cultivate positive thinking. Avoid being a couch potato, napping, and engaging in emotional eating. Create exciting ideas.

You can warm **baekan** by drinking warm beverages. Sip warm, pure water or tea and other warming drinks. Eat warming foods, such as spices, ginger, and lightly cooked, seasoned vegetables that grew in the sun. Avoid a diet of fatty and fried foods, sauces, milk soups, legumes, and root vegetables, such as potatoes, that grow in the ground. Wear warm clothes. If you have a **baekan** constitution, live and work in a warm, dry environment.

BALANCE AND IMBALANCE

How the Nyepa Interact

Proper functioning and interaction of the fifteen subdivisions of the *nyepa* produce seven body constituents during the process of digestion:

1. Nutritional essence from ingested foods and beverages gives rise to:
2. Blood that gives rise to:
3. Muscle that gives rise to:
4. Fat that gives rise to:
5. Bone that gives rise to:
6. Marrow that gives rise to:
7. Regenerative fluid, essential for health and conception.

The overall digestive process takes seven days. Beyond regenerative fluid, supreme vitality is the final product of this chain of syntheses. Supreme vitality resides primarily in the heart center but pervades the entire body to sustain life and promote vigor and radiance.

When the *nyepa* work together harmoniously, the body produces the seven body constituents and three waste products: feces, urine, and perspiration. Tibetan medicine calls the seven body constituents and three waste products the Ten Objects of Harming. Imbalance in **loong**, **tripa**, and **baekan** causes malfunctioning of the Ten Objects of Harming, which leads to suffering and disease.

Elaborate Network

The components of the body function through an elaborate network of nerves, blood vessels, energy channels, and other passages. These passages connect the external and internal parts of the body. They facilitate the storage and metabolism of nutrients essential for life. The seven bodily constituents function in seven passages. Excretion of the three waste products takes place through three passages. Food and lymph move through two passages.

The brain has five hundred channels of sensory functions that are responsible to perceive and grasp their respective objects. The heart has five hundred channels of memory functions that are responsible for clarity and development of consciousness. The navel has five hundred channels responsible for formation and development of the body. The genitals have five hundred channels responsible for reproduction. These channels, which exist above, below, and parallel to the navel, regulate all aspects of the body and are essential to sustain life.

Proper Alignment

Loong, **tripa**, and **baekan** continuously interact with each other. They are like a mobile hanging over a baby's crib. If you pull down one side of the mobile, the other side rises. Similarly, an out-of-balance energy can cause imbalance in the other two energies. If, for example, your **tripa** increases, your **baekan** and/or **loong** decrease.

You have fifteen subdivisions of *nyepa*, seven body constituents, and three waste products. To be happy and healthy, you must keep all twenty-five components in balance. In addition, your nerves, blood vessels, energy channels, and other passages must function well. Health results from proper alignment of all of these components in a dynamic state of equilibrium.

Disease results from a lack of alignment and disequilibrium in these components. If you do not maintain your three primary energies, they can harm your body and produce illness. Your *nyepa* can cause your seven body constituents and three waste products to malfunction. Disorders can develop in your nerves, blood vessels, energy channels, and other passages due to overflow, blockage, diversion, and disturbance.

Four Stages of Life

Between birth and death, you transition through four stages. You need appropriate energy to carry out the functions of each stage. Your health affects the age range during which you experience each stage. Maintaining good health may extend a particular stage. If you die prematurely, you must go through all four stages quickly. Table 4.1 lists the ideal time and prevalence of energy during each stage of life.

Table 4.1. The Four Stages of Life

Stage	Age	Prevalence of Energy
Child	Birth to about 20 years old	*Baekan*
Young adult	About 20 to 45 years old	*Tripa*
Adult	About 45 to 70 years old	*Tripa*
Elder	After age 70	*Loong*

During the first stage of life, *baekan* energy is highest. *Baekan* helps infants and children to grow, develop, sleep, and eat what they need. For children, this stage goes slowly. Usually, children are eager to grow up and enter the next stage.

Tripa energy is highest during young adulthood, the second stage, when sufficient energy is needed to transition from childhood to an adult life. *Tripa* decreases but still is elevated during mature adulthood, the third stage. Heat is required to produce energy for these active stages.

During the fourth stage, the elder period, *tripa* and *baekan* decrease and *loong* increases. Normally *loong* is highest in old age, particularly before death. Elevated *loong* counteracts being grounded. Then, ideally, *loong* promotes letting go and dying when mind and body are worn out.

MEDITATION: ALTERNATE NOSTRIL BREATHING

Daily meditation will help to keep your *nyepa* in balance. Meditation is a spiritual practice for becoming familiar with the mind. By doing Alternate Nostril Breathing, you will learn to focus your mind and create equilibrium. This meditation gives each side of the body equal time and strengthens the breath in the weaker nostril.

How to Meditate while Doing Alternate Nostril Breathing

- Sit or lie down comfortably with a straight back.
- Lower or close your eyes slightly and relax your mind and body.
- Breathe in a circular manner: Breathe through your nostrils, from your abdomen, slowly, deeply, evenly, with the in-breath the same length as the out-breath, and no break in between.
- Place your right thumb on your right nostril, your ring finger on your left nostril, and inhale through both nostrils.
- Use your thumb to close your right nostril; exhale slowly through your left nostril, and then inhale slowly through your left nostril.
- Use your ring finger to close your left nostril; exhale slowly through your right nostril, and then inhale slowly through your right nostril.
- This sequence constitutes one round; repeat for five more rounds.
- Focus on your breath; when the mind wanders away, bring it back to your breath.

Ordinarily, you don't breathe evenly through both nostrils all the time. Instead, one nostril closes, and you breathe through the other nostril for about ninety minutes. The closed nostril opens, the open nostril closes, and you breathe through the open nostril for about ninety minutes. You cycle back and forth every ninety minutes or so, depending on your health and circumstances.

Breathing through the right nostril stimulates the left brain. Breathing through the left nostril stimulates the right brain. During the few moments when your breathing shifts from one nostril to the other one, you are in balance and you breathe through both nostrils equally. You can use this automatic, natural process to treat insomnia.

Lie on your back in bed and relax. Do circular breathing as described above. Place your finger by one nostril and then the other one to determine which nostril is open and which one is closed. Turn on your side so that your open nostril is down, and your closed nostril is up, and breathe twenty-one times. Your open nostril will close, and your closed nostril will open. When your closed nostril opens, turn on your other side so that your open nostril is down, and your closed nostril is up, and breathe twenty-one times. Your open nostril will close, and your closed nostril will open. Focus on breathing in a circular manner while you continue this process of turning from side to side to open and close your nostrils until you fall asleep.

In summary, developing understanding of your three primary energies will help you to recognize when they are out of sync with your constitution. By being mindful, you will make informed choices to reverse this imbalance, or at least keep the imbalance from getting worse.

In the next chapter, you will learn more about your constitution. Understanding your true nature will help you to use your inherent characteristics as strengths, not weaknesses. You will develop appreciation and compassion for yourself and everyone else.

· 5 ·

Learn about Your Unique Nature

*T*ibetan medicine teaches that everyone is born with a unique combination of the three primary energies: *loong*, *tripa*, and *baekan*. *Nyepa* is the Tibetan term for the three primary energies. Your individual mixture of *nyepa* is called your true nature, your inborn constitution, or, simply, your constitution. The closest Western concept is DNA or inherited genetic code.

Wisdom traditions around the world teach "Know yourself." Tibetan medicine goes much deeper. To *really* know yourself, you must understand the energies comprising your constitution and how they affect you.

Your habitual way of responding results in large part from your constitution or home base. Your constitution determines to a great extent your body type, character, likes, dislikes, strengths, and weaknesses. You are healthy when the current percentages of your *loong*, *tripa*, and *baekan* are about the same as in your constitution. If you recognize who you *really* are, you will make choices that keep your *nyepa* in balance. You will choose your diet, behavior, friends, work, home, environment, and everything else to support your constitution.

This chapter challenges you to answer in-depth the question "Who *really* am I?" You will learn about the seven general constitutions of Tibetan medicine and how to live harmoniously with your unique constitution. The chapter ends with the beloved Tibetan meditation *Om Mani Padme Hum*. Meditating on and chanting this famous Sanskrit mantra cultivates compassion and wisdom that are vital for health and happiness.

WHO *REALLY* AM I?

The Seven General Constitutions of Tibetan Medicine

Tibetan medicine classifies constitutions into seven general types. Each type gets its name from the primary energy, or energies, that is dominant. *Loong, tripa,* or *baekan* dominates three constitutions. In three dual constitutions, *loong/tripa, loong/baekan,* or *tripa/baekan* are dominant. The seventh constitution consists of nearly equal percentages of *loong/tripa/baekan.*

The Seven General Constitutions of Tibetan Medicine

1. *Loong*: Movement energy dominates *tripa* and *baekan.*
2. *Tripa*: Hot energy dominates *loong* and *baekan.*
3. *Baekan*: Cold energy dominates *loong* and *tripa.*
4. *Loong/tripa* and *tripa/loong*: Movement and hot energies dominate *baekan.*
5. *Loong/baekan* and *baekan/loong*: Cold and movement energies dominate *tripa.*
6. *Tripa/baekan* and *baekan/tripa*: Hot and cold energies dominate *loong.*
7. *Loong/tripa/baekan* (rare constitution): All three energies are equal.

In all seven constitutions, the unique combination of *loong, tripa,* and *baekan* equals 100 percent. When one energy dominates, generally this energy makes up at least 50 percent of the constitution, and the other two energies together add up to 50 percent or less of the constitution. For a dual constitution, two energies each are about 40 percent, for a total of about 80 percent of the constitution, with lesser influence from the third energy.

For example, you have a *tripa* constitution if it is made up of about 60 percent *tripa,* 25 percent *baekan,* and 15 percent *loong.* You have a *loong/tripa* dual constitution if it consists of about 45 percent *loong,* 40 percent *tripa,* and 15 percent *baekan.* Your constitution is *loong/tripa/baekan* if you have about 33 percent of each *nyepa,* but this constitution is very rare. Most likely, you were born with one of the other six constitutions.

Only highly evolved individuals are born with equal percentages of *loong*, *tripa*, and *baekan*. This constitution gives them ready access to each primary energy in any situation. They can use all three energies to maintain mental and physical health. However, keeping each *nyepa* at about 33 percent is complicated. Few people are born with sufficient spiritual resources to maintain a *loong/tripa/baekan* constitution.

Keep Your Nyepa in Sync with Your Constitution

One or two primary energies likely dominate your constitution. To be happy and healthy, you need to focus on keeping your most influential energy or energies in balance. If, for example, you have a *tripa* constitution, you have ready access to *tripa* but not to *loong* or *baekan*. Therefore, you are most vulnerable to *tripa* imbalance and disease. A *tripa* imbalance is more serious for you than if you develop a *loong* and/or *baekan* disorder.

Similarly, if you have a *tripa/baekan* constitution, you are most influenced by *tripa* and *baekan* and less by *loong*. Keeping *tripa* and *baekan* in balance is challenging. When your *tripa* increases, your *baekan* likely will decrease. If you do what is cooling to decrease your *tripa*, your *baekan* may rise too high. You constantly need to make choices that keep *tripa* and *baekan* consistent with your constitution.

Even so, a dual constitution is preferable to a constitution dominated by one primary energy. If *tripa* and *baekan* dominate your constitution, you have ready access to both energies. Likewise, a *loong/tripa* constitution gives you ready access to *loong* and *tripa*. A *loong/baekan* constitution offers ready access to these energies.

When one primary energy goes out of balance, you are best off reversing the imbalance promptly. If not, the other two energies may go out of sync, too. Imbalance in all three *nyepa* results in complicated illnesses, such as autoimmune disorders, that are difficult to reverse. Bringing all of the *nyepa* into balance is challenging because they interact with each other.

Your Constitution Is Inborn

Ordinarily, your inborn nature remains the same all your life. Your constitution was established in your mother's womb by your consciousness, your karma, the constitution of your mother's ovum, the constitution of your father's sperm, and your mother's diet and behavior during pregnancy. For example, you likely have a *tripa* constitution if your consciousness, karma, mother's ovum, and father's sperm primarily were *tripa* and your mother indulged in a hot diet, behavior, and lifestyle when pregnant.

Before your conception, the afflictive nature of the *nyepa* already existed in your consciousness, karma, mother's ovum, and father's sperm. This symbiotic relationship is like poisonous parasites coexisting with a host that serves as the source of their survival. Knowing your true nature—your unique inborn constitution—will help you to take steps to enhance what is positive and counteract what is negative.

Your Three Primary Energies Rise and Fall

Your *nyepa* rise and fall throughout your life because of multiple influences. If, for example, you have a *tripa* constitution, *tripa* dominates *loong* and *baekan*. Even so, your *tripa* energy does not remain equally strong during your life. Your *tripa* rises and falls in the various stages of life, the seasons, and even a single day.

Ideally, *tripa* is low in childhood, high in young adulthood, decreasing but still elevated in mature adulthood, and low during the last stage of life. Moreover, *tripa* rises in the summer when the weather is hot and each day around noon and at midnight. Your *tripa* increases when you make choices that produce heat, such as getting angry, exercising vigorously, and eating spicy food. Your *nyepa*, desires, and perspective may alter, but you remain basically the same person.

Although your constitution ordinarily doesn't change, conditions of life bombard your *nyepa*, requiring continual adjustment. Negative thinking, stress, poor diet, unhealthy behavior, and variations in heat, cold, and weather disturb the *nyepa* and produce biochemical changes that promote suffering and disease. Some adjusting takes place automatically because of your inborn wisdom, but other regulation requires your conscious choice. Because health is order and disease is dis-order (lack of order), you need to become aware of any imbalance and promptly reverse it. Then, ideally, you will make choices that keep the current percentages of your three primary energies about the same as their percentages in your constitution.

Learning more about characteristics of the seven general constitutions will help you to identify yours and how to keep it in balance. As you read the following characteristics, figure out which ones fit you best. Discern who you *really* are, not the person you want to be. Consulting with someone who knows you well, such as your parent or partner, can help you to assess yourself accurately. Because you have all three *nyepa*, you exhibit some characteristics of each constitution, but one constitution describes you best.

LOONG CONSTITUTION: NATURE OF A VULTURE, CROW, AND FOX

Characteristics

If you have a ***loong*** constitution, you likely resemble a vulture, crow, and fox. Your facial features are sharp like a vulture. Your voice is harsh like a crow. You are sly like a fox, as you move from one location and experience to another one. ***Loong*** gives you characteristic physical traits, temperament, lifestyle, and vulnerabilities.

Your physical traits include being unusually tall or short with stooped shoulders and a bluish, dusty complexion for your gender and ethnic group. Your hair is thick, and your nails are brittle. You are delicate, weak, and thin, and you have difficulty gaining weight. Your joints are prominent and make crackling sounds when you move. You frequently yawn. Your thirst is irregular, your dry skin cracks easily. You seldom sweat and you vacillate between feeling hot or cold. Sometimes you are hungry, and other times you have no interest in food. Your tongue is red, dry, and rough, and your mouth is dry.

With a ***loong*** temperament, you likely are creative, fun, and spiritual, and you enjoy singing and dancing. You are passionate about music, art, games, debate, ideas, and projects. Your thoughts come rapidly and compete with each other. Because you like to talk, you often talk too much. You tend to be greedy, forgetful, "windy," unpredictable, unstable, unreliable, and restless. Anxious and worried, you ruminate about your problems. You like to be on the go. When quarrelsome, you can be rude. You don't want to plan, and you easily change your mind.

A *loong* constitution produces a characteristic lifestyle. You like to sit in the sun, but you dislike extreme heat and chilly, windy, frigid weather. Your preference is for fancy food with sweet, sour, and salty tastes. You have difficulty focusing, and you bounce from one activity to another one. Your finances tend to be unsound. You have trouble going to sleep, are a light sleeper, and easily awaken from sleep. Your sexual life is variable, and you have an active fantasy life. Because you use up your energy, you are prone to a short life span. You have a good sense of humor, you like to laugh, and you are fun to be around. Although you know many people, you don't feel close to them.

Because of *loong* vulnerabilities, you are supersensitive physically and emotionally. You are prone to developing stress-related disorders affecting your stomach, heart, blood vessels, and large intestine. Due to your irregular meals and digestive heat, you tend to have digestive difficulties. You are susceptible to developing addictions and mental health problems. When sick, you are nervous, and pains move around your body. You have irregular, hard, dry bowel movements and frequently are constipated.

Keep **Loong** in Balance

If you have a *loong* constitution, you need to keep the current percentage of your *loong* energy about the same as its percentage in your constitution. Maximize the strengths of *loong*. Transform the weaknesses of *loong* into benefits, or at least take steps to counteract them. To be happy and healthy, calm *loong* by eating an optimal diet, choosing an optimal lifestyle, and avoiding behaviors that cause *loong* to go out of balance.

You can calm *loong* by engaging in behavior that is grounding and warming. Walk in nature. Wear warm clothes. Live and work in warm, peaceful environments. Stay home and be quiet. Talk less and listen more. Limit your time on the phone and at your computer.

A *loong* optimal diet consists of warm, protein-rich, not-easily-digested foods, such as legumes and grains. Eat regular, warm, nutritious meals. Steer clear of cold foods and beverages such as ice cream and iced drinks. Consume dairy products if you can digest them. Add mild spices to food. Stay away from raw, acidic fruits and vegetables, such as tomatoes and green salads. Drink warm herbal tea. Avoid caffeine and other stimulants. If you tolerate alcohol, drink an occasional glass of wine but keep in mind that you are prone to addiction.

Choose an optimal lifestyle for your *loong* constitution. Decrease emotional stress. Sleep well at night. Listen to pleasant, calming music. Participate in harmonious conversations with friends and loved ones. Don't use mind-altering drugs. Respond immediately to every need of your mind and body. Avoid activities that cause *loong* to go out of balance.

TRIPA CONSTITUTION: NATURE OF A TIGER AND MONKEY

Characteristics

If you have a *tripa* constitution, your characteristics resemble a tiger and monkey. You are assertive and even aggressive like a tiger, and you have the energy of a monkey. *Tripa* gives you particular physical traits, temperament, lifestyle, and vulnerabilities.

Your *tripa* physical traits include a body that is muscular, well-proportioned, and medium in height and weight for your gender and ethnic group. You gain or lose weight easily. Your skin is light, and your hair tends to be sandy-colored, blond, or reddish for your ethnic group. In the sun, you easily burn, or your skin darkens, depending on your ethnicity. Your hair and skin are oily, your skin is hot and dry, and you have a slightly elevated body temperature. You are thirsty most of the time, and you sweat easily with foul-smelling perspiration. Your appetite, blood circulation, and digestive heat are good. You digest food quickly and frequently have loose stools. Your tongue has a thick, yellowish coat.

With a *tripa* temperament, you are bold, courageous, determined, and self-aware. Also you are prone to being jealous, proud, and stubborn. "Fiery," you quickly get angry, frustrated, and irritable under stress. You tend to be intelligent and have clear thinking. Your mind is quick, sharp, and focused. An ambitious, charismatic leader, you tend to be compelling and persuasive. You are good at initiating projects, setting goals, and working hard to achieve them.

Your *tripa* lifestyle provides moderate wealth. You enjoy mental and physical activities that are competitive, adventurous, athletic, impetuous, and daring. Your sex drive is good, and you are interested in sex. You tend to have a moderate-length life span, as long as you conserve your energy and don't try to do too much. Your preference is for cool, well-ventilated, dimly lit environments and sweet, bitter, astringent tastes.

Tripa has several vulnerabilities. You are susceptible to disorders that result from too much heat, which is why you easily get fevers, infections, inflammations, and skin rashes such as acne and psoriasis. Your most vulnerable organs are your liver, gallbladder, and small intestine. Because of heat, your hair tends to turn gray and you may get bald prematurely. You are prone to becoming addicted to alcohol.

Keep *Tripa* in Balance

If you have a *tripa* constitution, you need to keep the current percentage of your *tripa* about the same as its percentage in your constitution. Strengthen the benefits of *tripa*. Transform the weaknesses into assets, or at least keep them from creating obstacles for you. To be happy and healthy, cool *tripa*, eat an optimal diet, choose an optimal lifestyle, and avoid behaviors that cause *tripa* to go out of balance.

You can cool *tripa* by living in a moist, lukewarm climate. Stay out of the sun. Create cool, soothing spaces in which to live and work. Engage in activities that cool you down, rather than warm you up.

Ingesting an optimal diet cools a *tripa* constitution. Eat foods that cool you down, such as green leafy vegetables and cold salads. Ingest fruit of all kinds. Drink cool water and other cool beverages. Eat frozen foods, such as ice cream, in moderation.

Choose an optimal lifestyle for cooling *tripa*. Cultivate a peaceful mind. Decrease stress that heats you up. Engage in physical activities that are cooling. Take cool showers. Spend time by the water, surrounded by shady trees. Vacation in a cool, moist climate.

Avoid activities that cause *tripa* to go out of balance. Examples are ingesting a diet that produces heat: red meat, oil, fat, strong spices, coffee. Stay away from stressful mental work, multitasking, and doing too much. Don't exercise in a hot setting or drink too much alcohol.

BAEKAN CONSTITUTION: NATURE OF A LION AND ELEPHANT

Characteristics

If you have a *baekan* constitution, your characteristics resemble a lion and an elephant. You are strong like a lion and large, slow, and grounded like an elephant. *Baekan* gives you particular physical traits, temperament, lifestyle, and vulnerabilities.

Physical traits of a *baekan* constitution include a well-developed, sound, strong, cold body. You walk slowly and deliberately with an erect posture. For your gender and ethnic group, you have a heavy build; your complexion is pale; your hair is thick, dark, and wavy; and your skin is thick, soft, and smooth. You tend to produce excess mucus and get colds easily. Your bones and joints are not obvious because of being covered with flesh. You gain weight easily but have difficulty taking off the pounds. Because you have a strong endurance involving hunger and thirst, you can skip a meal without significant discomfort. Your digestion is slow, due to your low digestive heat and metabolic rate, and you feel heavy and bloated after eating. You have regular, solid bowel movements. Your tongue is smooth and has a white coat.

Your *baekan* temperament gives you a calm disposition, and you don't easily get ruffled. You tend to be kind, affectionate, peaceful, and tolerant. In challenging situations, you are resilient, your endurance is strong, and you avoid violence. You are forgiving, but when angry you may carry a grudge indefinitely. Your sexual interest is steady. You are likely to be friendly, considerate, altruistic, and generous. Although shy, you are loyal, noble, and obedient. With a *baekan* lifestyle, you tend to accumulate wealth and have sound finances. You are likely to live a long life because you conserve your energy and you sleep deeply. Your preference is for fancy, sweet food. Even though you dislike cold, you are able to tolerate extreme climates.

Baekan vulnerabilities include susceptibility to obesity, high cholesterol, respiratory infections, indigestion, diabetes, and kidney disorders. You tend to develop imbalance from too much cold and moisture, and then you experience increased mucus and swelling in your face, hands, legs, and feet. Your lungs, respiratory tract, kidneys, spleen, and stomach are your most vulnerable organs. You are prone to developing dementia, such as Alzheimer's disease.

Keep *Baekan* in Balance

If you have a *baekan* constitution, you need to keep your current percentage of *baekan* about the same as in your constitution. Maximize the advantages of *baekan*. Transform weaknesses into benefits, or at least keep them from undermining you. To be healthy and happy, warm *baekan*, eat an optimal diet, choose an optimal lifestyle, and avoid behaviors that cause *baekan* to go out of balance.

You can warm *baekan* by engaging in warm, dry activities. Regularly and vigorously walk and do other physical exercise. Wear clothes that keep you warm and dry. Safely spend time in the sun. Avoid being outside in cold, wet weather.

Eat a diet that warms *baekan*. Ingest spicy, warm foods and beverages, such as slightly cooked, nutritious, seasoned vegetables with herbs. Drink warm, nutritious beverages. For example, sip pure, boiled, slightly cooled water with lemon. Only eat when you are hungry. Avoid engaging in emotional eating. Ingest small portions to keep from gaining weight.

Choose an optimal lifestyle for warming *baekan*. Create a warm, dry environment in which to live and work. To boost your metabolism, increase your daily activity. Vacation in a warm, dry climate. Set goals and accomplish them on time.

Avoid activities that cause *baekan* to go out of balance. Stay away from activities that are moist and cool, like swimming in cool water. Cut back on fatty, fried foods; sugar; soups with a lot of liquid; bananas; and starchy vegetables such as legumes and root vegetables. Cultivate mindfulness so that you don't engage in emotional eating to anesthetize negative emotions. Instead uncover the mental poisons and transform them into wisdom.

DUAL AND TRIPLE CONSTITUTIONS

Dual Constitutions

You have a dual constitution if two *nyepa* dominate your third *nyepa*. A dual constitution causes you to manifest characteristics of both dominant energies. If, for example, you have a ***tripa/baekan-baekan/tripa*** constitution, you exhibit characteristics of both ***tripa*** and ***baekan***.

A dual constitution is preferable to a constitution dominated by one primary energy. With a dual constitution, you have ready access to both dominant energies, but you also must keep both energies in balance. To be healthy and happy, follow the recommendations above for both dominant energies and the guidelines for each dual constitution described below.

Loong/Tripa-Tripa/Loong Constitution

Your physical traits include being physically strong and full of energy. Your digestive heat is good, but you often have constipation. Although your body is hot, your hands and feet may be cold. You tend to develop inflammations, infections, fever, headaches, and dizziness.

You are self-aware and ambitious. However, you use up energy talking about yourself. Because you change your opinions, you make promises that you don't keep. You are prone to being restless, angry, and even aggressive.

Your optional diet and lifestyle consist of cool foods, beverages, activities, and environment. Live and work in cool settings. Cultivate a calm, cool mind. Stay away from the hot sun and a spicy diet. Avoid vigorous exercise, especially in a hot room or hot weather.

Loong/Baekan-Baekan/Loong Constitution

Your physical traits are a body that is slim, medium in size, and well built for your gender and ethnic group. Because your digestive heat is weak, you are prone to indigestion. You tend to have poor blood circulation and to develop neurological disorders.

Your temperament is cool, nervous, and changeable. You tend to be tolerant. Prone to lethargy and procrastination, you have difficulty focusing and getting things done on time.

To create an optimal diet and lifestyle, ingest warm foods and beverages. Eat small portions of nutritious foods at regular times. Live and work in warm environments. Engage in frequent, vigorous exercise. Avoid stimulants, such as caffeine.

Tripa/Baekan–Baekan/Tripa Constitution

This constitution gives you specific physical traits. You feel both hot and cold in your body. Even though you are physically active, you tend to be overweight.

Likewise, your temperament is both hot and cold. You may vary from getting things done to procrastinating. Generally, you are harmonious, and your manner is thoughtful. You tend to be trustworthy and steady. If upset, though, you can become fiery and aggressive.

To create an optimal diet and lifestyle, ingest a nutritious, lukewarm diet. Engage in activities moderately. Live and work in moderately warm environments. Avoid sunbathing and doing other activities in a hot room or the hot sun. Avoid spicy foods and beverages.

Loong/Tripa/Baekan Constitution

Only highly evolved individuals are born with nearly equal percentages of *loong*, *tripa*, and *baekan*. This epitome of harmony is characterized by ready access to all three *nyepa*. However, keeping *loong*, *tripa*, and *baekan* in balance is complicated and requires advanced ethical and spiritual understanding. To maintain balance, follow the above recommendations for each of the three primary energies and the guidelines below for this triple constitution.

Your physical and mental traits are flexible and resilient. Your mind tends to be healthy.

You set goals and meet them.

Your temperament is ideal. You practice self-compassion and universal compassion. Generous and optimistic, you don't easily become discouraged. You deal well with challenging situations and people.

You can create an optimal diet and lifestyle by living by *loong* recommendations if your digestive heat is changeable. When your digestive heat is strong, follow *tripa* guidelines. Go by *baekan* instructions if your digestive heat is sluggish. Choose friends, work, and environments that you enjoy. Be mindful of your needs and meet them appropriately.

MEDITATION: *OM MANI PADME HUM*

Whatever your constitution, you will benefit by cultivating self-compassion, compassion toward yourself. Treat yourself gently and lovingly. Accept who you *really* are. You will develop understanding of and gratitude for your constitution.

Practicing self-compassion fills your heart with universal compassion for everyone and everything. You become mindful of all of the suffering around you and ask, "What can I do to help?" As you evolve ethically and spiritually, you do your part to heal the world.

Infinite compassion is the means to cultivate wisdom, the ability to see things as they *really* are. To develop wisdom, meditate on and come to understand the interdependent, impermanent nature of all phenomena. Waking up to this reality is essential to make good choices that lead to happiness for yourself and others.

Meditating on and chanting the beloved Tibetan mantra *Om Mani Padme Hum* cultivates compassion and wisdom. This profound mantra has various interpretations. During teachings, His Holiness the 14th Dalai Lama gives a simple explanation:

- *OM* (pronounced *AUM*) represents impure body, mind, and speech due to the three mental poisons and ignorance about the nonexistence of an inherent self.
- *MANI* depicts Jewel, meaning infinite compassion developed from wisdom about the interdependent nature of all phenomena.
- *PADME* denotes wisdom, awareness of interdependence and the nonexistence of an intrinsic self.
- *HUM* illustrates union of compassion and wisdom.

Tibetans believe that meditating on and chanting this mantra purifies impure body, mind, and speech through the union of compassion and wisdom. Chanting this mantra for someone who is dying assists the person to let go and die peacefully. On the internet, you can hear how Tibetans pronounce *Om Mani Padme Hum.*

How to Meditate on Om Mani Padme Hum

- Sit comfortably on a straight-back chair, meditation cushion, or the floor; or lie flat on your back with your arms along your sides.
- Straighten your back and breathe deeply.
- Lower or partially close your eyes and relax. Engage in circular breathing: Breathe through your nostrils, from your abdomen, slowly, deeply, evenly, with the in-breath the same length as the out-breath, and no break in between.
- While breathing in a circular manner, chant the mantra *Om Mani Padme Hum,* or listen to someone else chanting the mantra.
- As you chant or listen, let go of the three mental poisons and flood your heart with compassion and wisdom.
- At the end of your meditation, keep your heart filled with compassion and wisdom.

In summary, this chapter asked the question "Who *really* are you?" Purifying the three mental poisons and cultivating compassion and wisdom help you to answer this question. By learning about your true nature—your inborn constitution—you come to appreciate what a fine person you are. You maximize your strengths and lessen your weaknesses.

The next chapter explains how to create a healthy mind. Healing negativity promotes happiness and optimal health. Developing spiritual immunity surrounds you with positive energy that offers protection from challenging people and situations.

· 6 ·

Create a Healthy Mind

According to Tibetan medicine, happiness is the purpose of life. Like everyone else, you have the right and responsibility to be happy. Happiness is a lasting, joyful state, not just temporary pleasure from sensory experiences such as eating a delicious meal. After your basic needs are met, your mental state is an essential factor in happiness. To be happy, you need to create a healthy mind.

You may think that happiness results from physical comfort and success. This option is expensive and unending. No matter how many possessions and accomplishments you accumulate, you won't feel like you have enough. A more effective, less expensive option is to train your mind to be healthy and happy in any situation.

A strength of Tibetan medicine is its profound understanding of the relationship between mind, health, and happiness. Research validates this ancient, timely wisdom, as reviewed in chapter 15. Studies have found that healing negativity and practicing compassion positively affect mind and body. You are as happy as you choose to be.

Understanding the nature of mind is crucial. You jeopardize your health and happiness if you are ignorant about the fundamental reality of mind. A false view of who you *really* are is called *ma-rig-pa* (ignorance) in Tibetan.

This chapter gives an overview of Tibetan medicine's teachings about the nature of mind and why the three mental poisons produce suffering and dis-ease (lack of ease). You will learn how to heal negativity and develop spiritual immunity. The chapter ends with Mindfulness Meditation to help you create a healthy mind.

WHAT IS MIND?

Gross Mind and Subtle Mind

As a human being, you were born with two kinds of mind: gross mind and subtle mind. Your gross mind can only access conventional knowledge: what is impermanent, material, and typically known. Subtle mind can access ultimate reality, seeing things as they *really* are.

Gross mind, without subtle mind, lacks wisdom. Subtle mind, without gross mind, is too abstract for everyday decisions. If you only use your gross, logical mind, you are likely to reach wrong conclusions. Ideally, your subtle mind provides a wise vision for your life, and your gross mind carries it out.

A bird can fly in the sky and see the bigger picture, as well as return to the ground to get food to eat. Like a bird flying overhead, your subtle mind offers insight about your relationship to the cosmos. Through your subtle mind, you intuit answers to the important questions of life: Why am I here? Can I be healthy and happy? Is there a right way for me to live and die? How can I live with meaning and integrity? By training your gross mind, you can use the wisdom of your subtle mind to make healthy choices about everyday life.

If you choose to learn about your subtle mind, you may think that you must focus on your thoughts, emotions, interpretations, reactions, experiences, sensitivities, desires, and stories. You may assume that your subtle mind is your state of consciousness at any moment in time. Or you may define your subtle mind as the stimulus behind your thoughts, the total of everything in your brain. These assumptions and definitions are incorrect. If you base your investigation on them, you make the mistake of *ma-rig-pa* or ignorance. The activities of gross mind hide subtle mind.

Subtle mind is clear, perfect, and free. Simple and natural, subtle mind can't be complicated, corrupted, or stained. Subtle mind is primordial, pure, pristine awareness. Mere words and pictures can't describe subtle mind. Instead of being limited to only one individual, subtle mind is the true nature of everything, knowledge of knowledge itself. Subtle mind is intelligent, awake, intuitive, and creative.

Leading a busy, stressful life interferes with recognizing your subtle mind. You may catch glimpses, though, just as clouds shift to reveal the shining sun. Subtle mind is your inner wisdom and teacher. When your vision clouds over, subtle mind can guide you back to your true self. Accessing your subtle mind requires diminishing your gross mind so that it no longer covers up your subtle mind.

By becoming mindful of your subtle mind, you evolve ethically and spiritually. As you develop awareness, you accept who you *really* are. You treat yourself and others with compassion, and then you are less likely to behave in harmful ways.

Through meditation, you can become familiar with your subtle mind. The traditional meditative pose is to sit cross-legged, like an unshakable mountain. A mountain naturally is at ease, no matter how much wind batters it, rain and snow fall on it, and dark clouds swirl around its peak. During meditation, let your mind rise and soar like a bird. You will realize that your subtle mind is ageless, radiant, and fathomless. To learn more about the subtlest mind, read Tibetan Buddhism's Highest Yoga Tantra.

Mind and the Three Mental Poisons

Suffering begins with a self-centered mental attitude. Self-centeredness results from a lack of understanding about the fundamental reality of who you *really* are. This egotistical perspective is based on the false belief that you exist as an independent being. Self-obsessed, you focus on your own needs at the expense of others. Rather than recognize this ignorance, you think you have an accurate self-perception.

An ignorant, egotistical perspective leads to the three mental poisons: (1) greed, attachment, and desire; (2) anger, hostility, and aggression; and (3) delusion, confusion, and closed-mindedness. These afflictive emotions stimulate inappropriate behavior in body, mind, and speech and cause the subsequent birth of *loong*, *tripa*, and *baekan*.

The three mental poisons result from an egotistical perspective. If, for example, you are attached to someone, you feel angry if the person doesn't behave the way you want. You are deluded about your opinion being right because your ego has so much at stake. By pressuring the person to follow your wishes, you cause conflict in the relationship.

When attached to your ego, you fail to see things as they *really* are. Your gross mind, conditioned by the three mental poisons, keeps you from seeing reality. Confused, you can't think clearly, and you let negativity dictate your life. Not knowing anything different, you assume that this unhealthy mental state is normal.

Besides upsetting your peace of mind and relationships, the three mental poisons cause havoc in your body. Any one of the three mental poisons can change your body's biochemistry directly or indirectly. Your five elements, the source of your existence, go out of balance. Dis-equilibrium in your **earth, water, fire, air,** and **space** cause your *loong*, *tripa*, and *baekan* to rise too high, fall too low, and/or become disturbed. If not reversed, this dysfunction gives rise to pathology.

You can end this cycle by uncovering and healing self-centeredness—the source of negativity. If you aren't attached to your ego, the three mental poisons won't arise. A non-egotistical, compassionate, wise perspective tames them when they do appear.

Mind-Body Relationship

The dynamic relationship between mind and body can be difficult to comprehend. Here is an example to help you understand. When you get angry at someone, you trigger in your mind and body a fight or flight response: You want to fight or run away. Your initial response and subsequent reactions boost your energy to deal with the perceived threat from the person at whom you are angry. Your neurons fire, and adrenaline, noradrenaline, and cortisol are released into your bloodstream.

The firing of your neurons and release of chemicals cause dramatic changes. Your blood pressure, blood sugar, and heart rate increase. You breathe in a shallow, erratic manner. Your immune system becomes depressed.

Even if the situation isn't *really* an emergency, your **fire** element and *tripa* energy produce more heat than needed. Elevated heat gives rise to heat-related disorders, such as high blood pressure, headaches, gastrointestinal upset, autoimmune diseases, inflammations, infections, skin rashes, and metabolic disorders. Eventually, *tripa* imbalance causes *loong* and *baekan* imbalance, leading to more dysfunction.

NEGATIVE THINKING, SUFFERING, AND DISEASE

Negative Thinking and Suffering

Mind is the source of health and happiness, as well as disease and suffering. You undermine yourself if you believe that engaging in the three mental poisons will make you happy. Dissatisfied, agitated, egocentric thinking upsets mind and body. Under the influence of negative thinking, you make poor choices with disastrous results.

The more negative your thinking, the more you suffer. You fail to understand the effects of your behavior. For example, you may wish to harm someone you think hurt you. Getting revenge may bring momentary relief. Later, feelings of alienation and unease arise, leading to more negativity. Rather than see the connection between your negativity and suffering, you blame others for life not going the way you want. You are like an alcoholic who doesn't recognize the destructiveness of inappropriate drinking.

The three mental poisons are deceiving because they seem to offer satisfaction. Coming in the guise of a protector, negativity gives boldness and strength. At the same time, negativity destroys a precious quality: the capacity for discriminative awareness. The three mental poisons take away the ability to make healthy choices and discern likely outcomes. Decisions made under the influence of negativity later are a source of regret.

The three mental poisons encourage the assumption that appearances are the same as reality. When, for example, you are angry, you focus on the person's negative traits and see them as permanent. You forget that this individual is a suffering human being who wants to be happy, just as you do. If you let go of anger and view this person in a positive light, you will make better choices about how to deal well with the situation in a manner that produces good consequences.

The more you give in to the three mental poisons, the less space you have for compassion, wisdom, and successful conflict resolution. Unrestrained negativity increases like a river that floods when snow melts. Mental poisons enslave the mind. If you indulge in negativity, you become accustomed to it. You habituate yourself to unethical behavior.

Negative Thinking and Disease

The impact of unethical behavior registers deep within. You may mistakenly deny and suppress the three mental poisons, as when you hide anger and present a facade of self-control. However, this lack of honesty leads to more negativity. Eventually, unethical behavior bursts out physically and/or emotionally when you can't contain it any longer.

As the negative cycle continues, you become oblivious to the impact of your behavior. Research reviewed in chapter 15 confirms that negativity is disastrous for both mind and body. By engaging in the three mental poisons, you sabotage yourself and others. Stressed-out, you don't breathe properly. Your cells become sick from a lack of oxygen and buildup of toxins. Because of the karma you accumulate from unethical behavior, you bring back more negativity on yourself.

Positive behavior arises from positive intentions, emotions, and thoughts. In contrast, negative thinking and acts result from the three mental poisons. Positive behavior is ethical, compassionate, wise, right, and virtuous. Negative behavior is unethical, violent, unwise, wrong, and lacking in virtue. Intention is most important. An act is unethical when the desire to cause harm motivates a seemingly positive act.

The way to be happy is to heal negative reactions to life's challenges. Transform the mental poisons into positive behavior. When you *really* understand the true nature of mind, you will train yourself to behave in a manner that creates health and happiness, not suffering and disease, regardless of your circumstances.

HEAL NEGATIVITY

Mindfulness

The three mental poisons have an excellent quality: You can transform them into positive behavior. You can reverse the process of the mental poisons governing your mind and disrupting your life. Conversely, be mindful of when positivity shifts into unethical behavior.

You will tame the three mental poisons by understanding that all phenomena are interconnected. A wave is not distinct from the ocean but part of the ocean. Similarly, you are not a separate, independent being but completely dependent upon everything around you. All phenomena are interconnected and interdependent. You affect others and they affect you. Narcissism, focusing on yourself, creates suffering, not happiness.

Take a moment to imagine how much simpler and joyful life is if you heal the three mental poisons. Your self-esteem rises. When you try to sleep, negative thoughts don't keep you awake. You no longer feel insecure when your colleague gets a job or pay raise that you want. If someone fails to appreciate your opinions, you don't spend precious time and energy clinging to your ego and trying to save face.

To heal negativity, develop mindfulness about what you do, what you think, and what you say. Pay close attention to your body, mind, and speech. Rather than allow the mental poisons to upset your balance, figure out where they come from. Think like a scientist who collects and analyzes data and then draws appropriate conclusions. Investigate the source of even your slightest negativity and let it go.

This task is not easy. For example, hatred is a strong emotion when fully developed. In its beginning stages, though, you may notice only subtle aversion. Gaining insight into yourself is a lifelong task. Unless you undertake this investigation, you won't see how to make positive changes. The more you develop virtuous qualities, the more you will increase their influence and the happier you will be.

The process of healing the mental poisons doesn't mean denying or suppressing them. Face up to what troubles you. Recognize and heal your broken heart. Otherwise, negativity will express itself in mental and/or physical disease. Similarly, an infected wound must be cleaned before it heals. Left untended, infection is poisonous.

Befriend your mind, instead of avoiding it. Bring into your consciousness what is unconscious. Work with this content to root out and heal negativity. Analyze the conditions that result in happiness and which ones don't. Then make choices that increase happiness and decrease suffering.

The next time you feel strong attachment or aversion, recognize that egotistical thoughts are bothering you. Change your focus from yourself to others. Practicing compassion toward yourself, and others will cause your own problems to diminish. As you let go of the three mental poisons, you will have an easier time generating positive emotions and behaviors. By transforming your thinking, you transform your life.

Ethical Behavior

After your basic needs are met, you have everything you need for happiness. The key is your interpretation, not the situation. For example, you may get upset if you are caught in the rain, but you enjoy taking a shower in your bathroom. You get wet in each situation, but your attitude differs because of your interpretation.

Thoughts, emotions, and events are the source of anger and despair, but also of ethical and spiritual evolution. You choose how to interpret life's challenges. If you steer clear of negative thinking, you are more likely to make healthy choices that bring back positive consequences. Good decisions don't solve everything, but they avoid making things worse. You cultivate compassion and wisdom by dealing well with whatever occurs.

Even in difficulties, habituate yourself to ethical behavior. Behave with integrity by living up to your best values. Create meaning by seeing your life as part of a bigger, purposeful picture. It's up to you how to let challenging circumstances affect you.

You can heal your mind by expressing sincere regret and making amends for your harmful behavior. Most important, make amends to yourself because you have hurt yourself the most. Avoid negative self-talk, such as saying, "I'm not good enough!" Instead, treat yourself lovingly and gently as you do a newborn baby.

To fully heal negativity, root out the three mental poisons. When they arise, just let them pass through your mind like clouds in the sky. Letting go of negativity keeps it from lodging in your mind. If you express afflictive emotions, you run the risk of overreacting and causing harm. Instead of responding negatively, take a time out. Once you regain your balance, you will make better choices about how best to deal with the situation.

You can heal the mental poison of greed, attachment, and desire by meditating on and coming to accept impermanence. All phenomena are in flux. Everyone's cells continuously change. Trying to make things permanent doesn't work. As in Mountain and Willow yoga postures, sometimes you need to be strong and tall like a mountain. Other times, flexibility like a willow tree is best. Accepting, not fighting, impermanence will help you to determine when to stand firm and when to adapt.

Meditate on and cultivate compassion to heal the mental poison of anger, hostility, and aggression. Recognize that other people wish to be free of suffering but often feel helpless to make changes. Rather than be resigned to negativity, choose the attitude that you can heal suffering. You can transform your sadness, fear, depression, and contempt. As you develop compassion, your capacity for cruelty and delight in other people's misfortunes will subside.

You can heal the mental poison of delusion, confusion, and closed-mindedness by meditating on and developing wisdom. Take off the blinders and see things as they *really* are, not as you want them to be. Wisdom means to wake up and to see everything, even what you don't want to see. Yoga postures produce various views: up, down, sideways, backwards. Doing the same with your thinking will help you to cultivate wisdom. If you analyze a situation from many perspectives, you will make better choices than if you lock yourself into only one viewpoint.

Challenging Individuals and Situations

At first, you may have difficulty behaving with compassion toward individuals you think have treated you badly. If so, avoid them until you become stronger mentally. Develop spiritual and emotional capabilities to practice compassion instead of anger. Surround yourself with people you enjoy and who encourage you to be positive.

Set limits with anyone who abuses you emotionally and/or physically. Proper boundaries are essential in all relationships. If someone threatens you, you'd better run away rather than get hurt. Your anger at the person may be justified. Keep in mind, though, that negativity increases if anger becomes personal and turns into malice. Create healthy attachments and avoid codependency, too much reliance on another person.

If you find offense at people who behave badly, you get hurt twice: first by their actions and then even more by your reactions to them. You can choose whether to take this conflict lightly or try to get even. When you become obsessed with how you were harmed, you are likely to develop anxiety, insomnia, miserable days and nights and, eventually, disease. By letting hurt fester, you will create an unhealthy, unhappy life.

When people behave in harmful ways, they are engaging in the three mental poisons and suffering as a result. If you treat them with negativity, you cause more suffering for yourself and them, and then they might behave even worse. Like you, they want to be happy, but they don't realize they are sabotaging themselves and creating suffering. You can't figure out their motives. Instead, recognize that the three mental poisons result from a vast, complex web of interrelated causes and conditions.

Yes, it's easy to care for your friends and dislike individuals who offend you. If your attitude changes, though, you may see your friends as enemies and your enemies as friends. Attitudes do change. Don't treat people according to how they treat you. Hostility will not disturb you if you train yourself to behave kindly toward everyone.

When someone harms you, tolerance will give you the strength to keep from engaging in the three mental poisons. Then, during adversity, you will remain unperturbed. Instead of reacting negatively, you will forgive the person.

One of the hardest tasks in life is to forgive. Forgiving doesn't necessarily mean to forget, reconcile, condone, deny, or excuse unethical behavior. Instead, forgiveness means to drop the burden of resentment and forgo revenge. You don't let negativity take over your mind and life.

Forgiveness helps you to move forward and increase your optimism. You aren't stuck in the past. Forgiveness lessens your suffering and adds deeper meaning to life. If you train yourself to forgive, you see more clearly how to avoid harmful situations. Forgiveness gives you the vision to reach out and help other individuals who have experienced hurt and a broken heart.

That's why nonviolence is essential. Avoid violence, even if someone is mean to you. Don't return harm for harm, or you will bring back violence on yourself. You will cope well with adversity by doing your part to change systems and situations that perpetuate violence. Partner with others to create a more compassionate, just world.

Do everything in your power to resolve conflict. If you can't change a challenging situation, though, you can learn to accept it. Worrying about what you can't change is a waste of precious time and energy and makes things worse. Often, the most ethical and spiritual growth occurs during times of great difficulty. By cultivating a positive perspective, you become stronger, not weaker. Challenges open your eyes to reality and help you to treat yourself and others with compassion.

Step-by-Step Patience

Changing your thinking from negative to positive isn't a quick fix. Buddhism teaches two different methods for training the mind to reach enlightenment. One approach is spontaneous insight. The other perspective is to train the mind step-by-step. In the eighth century, the Simultaneists and the Gradualists held a debate at *Samye*, the first Tibetan Buddhist monastery in Tibet, to determine the right path.

According to tradition, the Chinese *Chan* (Zen) master, Ho-sheng Mo-ho-yen, headed the Simultaneists. The Simultaneists assumed that meditative practice should consist primarily of thought cessation. They taught that stopping any kind of mental activity induces a simultaneous or instantaneous realization of awakening. For them, meditative insight alone was sufficient to achieve awakening. They considered the practice of compassion to be superfluous, or even obstructive to meditative insight.

On the other side of the debate, Kamalasila, a Buddhist from India, led the Gradualists. They viewed human thought as an instrument for developing compassion. Cultivating compassion, they asserted, was an essential component of ethical and spiritual evolution. They advocated a step-by-step approach, not instantaneous enlightenment. Each stage of growth, they claimed, was the foundation for the next one.

The Gradualists prevailed over the Simultaneists in Tibet. Since then, Tibetan medicine has advocated gradual, careful progression from one stage to the next. Training the mind requires step-by-step patience, rather than seeking emotional highs, mystical experiences, and fast spiritual growth.

When people treat you badly, your first instinct may be to get even. Tibetan medicine encourages a calm, generous response. If you hate them, they are likely to hate you. Develop gratefulness that they offer a precious opportunity to root out the three mental poisons. Treating them with kindness will help you to defuse the situation.

Shantideva,[1] an eighth-century Buddhist monk and scholar in India, taught that suffering arises from the longing for personal happiness, whereas happiness results from wanting others to be happy. He wrote a prescription for joy:

> And now as long as space endures, as long as there are beings to be found, may I continue likewise to remain to drive away the sorrows of the world (169).

DEVELOP SPIRITUAL IMMUNITY

What Is Spiritual Immunity?

Creating a happy, healthy mind consists of more than healing the three mental poisons and behaving ethically. Tibetan medicine advocates developing spiritual immunity—positive energy—to protect you from challenging individuals and situations. Spiritual immunity keeps you from sliding down the slippery slope of negativity.

A healthy physical immune system is essential for the body to prevent and heal disease. Likewise, spiritual immunity helps you to create a healthy mind and safeguard you from the three mental poisons, or at least diminish their effect. Cultivating positive energy in your mind, body, and environment thwarts negativity.

If your physical immune system functions properly, it detects a wide variety of foreign agents, such as viruses and bacteria, and distinguishes them from your own tissues. Similarly, a healthy spiritual immune system identifies mental poisons and neutralizes them. Often, negativity starts small and is difficult to identify until it becomes full-blown. You can create a strong spiritual immune system by developing mindfulness of your thoughts, even the very beginning of a thought. Train your mind to distinguish the mental poisons from positive thinking, and promptly let go of any negativity.

The Four Immeasurables

You can develop spiritual immunity by practicing Buddhism's Four Immeasurables.[2] Cultivating these virtues will help you to root out the three mental poisons. You will create a healthy mind and behavior. Table 6.1 describes the Four Immeasurables.

When other people mistreat you, respond with loving-kindness, compassion, empathetic joy, and equanimity. Practice the Four Immeasurables as a philosophical stance, not feelings that come and go. Then you won't use up precious energy deciding how to react. Train yourself to behave kindly toward everyone all the time

Kindness comes from the root "of the same kind." People who challenge you aren't "the other." They and you are of the same species. Everyone is made of the same five elements and three primary energies.

Table 6.1. Cultivate the Four Immeasurables

The Four Immeasurables	Definition	Action to Take	Your Resulting Behavior
Loving kindness	Heartfelt yearning for you and others to experience happiness and its causes.	Realize that everyone wants to be happy and that you are "of the same kind" as others.	You see Buddha-Nature, divine qualities, in yourself and other people.
Compassion	Heartfelt yearning for you and others to become free of suffering and its causes.	Recognize that you and others want to be free of suffering, but too often engage in the three mental poisons.	You ask kindly, "What can I do to help?"
Empathetic Joy	Delight in your own and other peoples' virtue, happiness, and success.	Turn your focus from yourself to others; let go of envy and cynicism.	You celebrate your own and other peoples' virtue, happiness, and success.
Equanimity	Impartiality; mindfulness without attraction or aversion.	Avoid being ruled by your passions, likes, and dislikes.	You behave calmly, even in challenging circumstances.

By cultivating the Four Immeasurables, you transform yourself and create healthy relationships.

Peaceful Mind, Body, and Life

Tibetan medicine has other advice for how to develop spiritual immunity and protect yourself from negativity. Take responsibility for your behavior. Think before you say anything and then speak wisely. Kindly state your perspective without dishonesty and arrogance. Listen to other people, but don't simply accept what they assert is true. Instead, investigate their claims and avoid being misled.

Cultivate healthy relationships with your family, friends, neighbors, colleagues, members of your communities, and everyone else you know. Repay the kindnesses that others do for you. Be true to your word and fulfill your commitments.

Protect yourself from people who behave in ways that are egotistical, deceitful, jealous, cruel, and unstable. Abstain from disclosing your secrets to them. To avoid regrets later, move ahead cautiously. Don't cede power to individuals who will do you wrong and even overpower you. Avoid overestimating and underestimating them.

Behave with moderation, instead of going from one extreme to the other. Think ahead. Rather than procrastinate, set goals and accomplish them within a reasonable time frame. Increase your knowledge and experience. Avoid boasting about your education, possessions, accomplishments, and anything else.

Cultivate contentment. Even so, diligently accumulate enough wealth to meet your own needs and avoid being dependent on others. In this way, you can function as an autonomous moral agent, rather than be controlled by someone else. However, be careful not to become obsessed with success. Don't focus on guarding your possessions from others, but give generously to individuals in need.

Even strive to help people who try to hurt you. Remain calm in the face of aggression. Adopt a generous attitude without any sense of stinginess. Consider the needs of others as being equal to your own needs.

Be mindful of your dreams, especially if they occur during the early morning *loong* period. Your dreams provide insight about your life and what is in your mind. A positive dream suggests health and happiness. Meditating will help you to learn from disturbing dreams and avoid negative influences. You are less likely to experience troubling dreams when you calm your mind, body, and life.

The more you heal the three mental poisons and strengthen your spiritual immune system, the more you interpret life from a positive perspective. You no longer take difficulties so seriously, but you see the humor in them. Obstacles that previously felt overwhelming now seem more manageable.

You experience peace that is unaffected by the inevitable ups and downs of life. Your relationships become smooth. You value others, and you feel valued by them. With clear thinking, you reach out to help others and contribute to the whole.

MINDFULNESS MEDITATION

Mindfulness Meditation will help you to create a healthy mind. Mindfulness means to be fully present in the moment, rather than be stuck in the past or future. By doing this meditation regularly, you become increasingly aware of what is in your mind. You transform the three mental poisons into satisfaction, compassion, and wisdom, and you develop spiritual immunity.

Tibetan medicine draws an analogy between the mind and a bird. No matter how high the bird soars in the sky, its shadow remains on the ground. Similarly, the purpose of life is to rise to your best self and create health and happiness for yourself and others. If you are shadowed by ignorance, however, you can't free yourself from suffering and disease.

Mindfulness Meditation removes ignorance by increasing your awareness of your body, mind, speech, and everything else. Mindfulness doesn't get you to be different from who you are at this moment, but to be who you *really* are. Eliminating mental poisons uncovers the natural calmness and harmony of your subtle mind.

You can do Mindfulness Meditation anywhere. For example, you can sit mindfully in the traditional cross-legged, lotus position on the floor or ground. When you attend a meeting or class, you can sit mindfully in a chair. You can lie mindfully in bed before getting up in the morning and going to sleep at night. Walk mindfully in a nature center or around your neighborhood. Mindfully choose, eat, and digest a healthy diet. Practice mindfulness while washing dishes and cleaning your home.

How to Do Mindfulness Meditation

- Sit comfortably on a straight-back chair, a meditation cushion, or the floor, or lie flat on your back with your arms along your sides.
- Straighten your back, breathe deeply, lower or close your eyes, and relax.
- Breathe in a circular manner, through your nostrils, from your abdomen, slowly, deeply, evenly, with your in-breath the same length as your out-breath, and no break in between.
- When you are deeply relaxed, focus on your breath or an object that is comfortable for you, or slowly count to ten over and over.
- Simply observe and let go of whatever arises in your mind, without attachment, judgment, or direction.
- Try to stay focused even though you experience myriad thoughts and emotions.
- Gently bring your focus back when your thoughts wander away from meditation.

After completing Mindfulness Meditation, continue breathing in a circular manner throughout the day and evening. Reflect on what you learned about yourself during your meditation. Bring mindfulness into your everyday life 24/7.

You not only have the resources to create a healthy mind, but you have the potential to evolve to a higher level of health and happiness. You can become fully awake, a state called enlightenment. The next chapter explains how to create an enlightened mind.

· 7 ·

Create an Enlightened Mind

$\mathscr{T}$ibetan medicine, the ancient science of healing from Tibet, is based on ancient observations, principles, and theories of the mind-body connection. These teachings are explained in the *Four Tantra* of the *Gyueshi*, the fundamental text of Tibetan medicine. The *Gyueshi* draws heavily from Tibetan Buddhism, the branch of Buddhism that flourished in Tibet. Tibetan medicine is one of the greatest legacies of Tibetan Buddhism. The *Gyueshi* is attributed to Shakyamuni Buddha, the historical Buddha. Learning about Tibetan Buddhism is essential to understand and apply Tibetan medicine.

Tibetan Buddhism is a philosophy, psychology, science of the mind, and religion. You will benefit from the philosophy, psychology, and science of the mind, whether or not you follow the religion. These teachings, which complement other wisdom traditions, are life transforming, regardless of your values, beliefs, or religion. You learn how to create *bodhicitta*, a Sanskrit term for the mind of enlightenment, and evolve into a *bodhisattva*, a Sanskrit term for someone devoted to compassion and wisdom. Eventually, you can become fully awake, a joyful state called Buddhahood or enlightenment.

This chapter gives an overview of Tibetan Buddhist philosophy, psychology, and science of the mind underlying Tibetan medicine. The chapter describes the Four Noble Truths and Eightfold Path of Ethics. Next, the chapter explains Buddhist concepts: impermanence, emptiness, dependent origination, interconnectedness, and universal compassion. The chapter ends with a meditation on the Medicine Buddha, the healing form of the Buddha that symbolizes Tibetan medicine and an enlightened mind.

BUDDHISM: BEYOND RELIGION

The Buddha

Buddhism was founded on the teachings of Siddhartha Gautama. According to tradition, he was born in 563 BCE in what is now Nepal. Because his father was king of the region, he seemed to have everything: social standing, a wife and child, good looks, wealth, and the throne he would inherit. Despite this luxury, he abandoned his life as a prince to find a way out of universal suffering and to seek enlightenment.

During the next six years, Siddhartha Gautama went through three stages. First, he studied with two of the foremost Hindu teachers of the day. Next, he joined a group of ascetics, after which he concluded that asceticism does not lead to freedom from suffering. Finally, he engaged in rigorous thought and meditation.

Sensing that a breakthrough was near, he sat down under a bodhi tree in Bodh Gaya, India. He vowed not to get up until he reached enlightenment. One morning, Siddhartha was gone and replaced by Shakyamuni Buddha, the historical Buddha. His followers called him the Buddha, meaning the Awakened One.

For the next forty-five years, the Buddha taught both women and men of all castes. The Buddha advocated the Middle Way between the extremes of indulgence and asceticism. He explained that everyone has the potential to wake up and become a Buddha, someone who sees things as they *really* are. The Buddha's followers wanted to know who he *really* was. They asked him if he was a god, a saint, or an angel. "No," the Buddha replied, "I am awake!"

Scholars believe that the Buddha lived and taught primarily in the eastern part of ancient India sometime between the sixth and fourth centuries BCE. Other world-famous teachers also lived during that time period: Hebrew prophets in Israel; Socrates, Plato, and Aristotle in Greece; Vyasa and other yogis in India; and Confucius and Lao Tzu in China. Their writings about ethics have similarities to the Buddha's teachings.

The Buddha's Teachings

According to the Buddha, you, like everyone else, want to be happy and avoid suffering. Happiness isn't accidental but the result of a balanced life and peaceful relationships. Informed choices transform imbalance into harmony. Through ethics and meditation, you can cultivate compassion and wisdom and create an enlightened mind.

Ethics, spirituality, healing, and happiness are interrelated, the Buddha taught, rather than being separate disciplines. Ethical behavior means to behave with compassion and wisdom toward all beings. Growing spiritually results from recognizing your interconnectedness with all phenomena. Behaving ethically and growing spiritually are essential for health and happiness.

Ethical behavior and spiritual growth create a healthy mind, the Buddha said. Moreover, they also generate *bodhichitta*. This Sanskrit word means the spontaneous wish to attain Buddhahood (enlightenment) for the benefit of all beings. *Bodhichitta* nurtures a mind that is becoming enlightened, and vice versa.

The Buddha taught that these teachings are medicine for the mind. If you engage in the three mental poisons and make unhealthy lifestyle choices, you are mistaken about how to be happy. You can't heal your mind unless you first acknowledge your suffering.

Other wisdom traditions from India use the Sanskrit term *Dharma*. In Buddhism, *Dharma* refers to the Buddha's teachings and subsequent commentaries. *Dharma* can be taught, but your heart and mind must be open to receive the teachings.

A three-pot analogy describes faults that keep you from understanding *Dharma*. If you are like an upside-down pot, *Dharma* falls out, and you can't benefit from the teachings. You can't remember *Dharma* when you are like a leaky pot. *Dharma* goes in one ear and out the other one. When you harbor resentment and hurt, you are like a pot with poison. You reinterpret *Dharma* to suit your purposes and contaminate the teachings.

Buddhism

The term Buddha refers to the historic prince, a human being. Buddhists are individuals who follow his teachings. The term Buddha has a deeper meaning, though. Buddha refers to anyone who has completely awakened from ignorance and has opened to the vast potential of wisdom. Awareness is both the path and the goal. You become a Buddha when you bring an end to your suffering, see things as they *really* are, and create lasting peace and joy.

Buddhism is classified into two major branches: Theravada and Mahayana. Theravada Buddhism, written in the Pali language, is viewed as the Buddha's root teachings. Theravada is practiced primarily in Sri Lanka, Cambodia, Thailand, Laos, and Myanmar (Burma). Mahayana Buddhism consists of the Pali Canon and later writings in Sanskrit. Mahayana is practiced in India, Tibet, China, Korea, Japan, Vietnam, Bhutan, Indonesia, and other countries. Theravada emphasizes personal enlightenment, whereas the Mahayana ideal is to become a *Bodhisattva*. Increasingly, both branches of Buddhism are being practiced in the West.

In Buddhism, God is not an anthropomorphic being but all the conscious energy in the universe. As a manifestation of this life force, you are responsible to help create a more compassionate, just world, rather than wait for a messiah to do this work. Buddhism doesn't require blind faith. Instead, investigate your thoughts, feelings, and actions. Set aside teachings that don't make sense and look at them later. Perhaps then you will find them to be justifiable.

The term Buddhism is misleading if it focuses on the historic person, Shakyamuni Buddha. The Tibetan term for Buddhism is *Nang choe*, which literally means "inner nature or nature of mind." Tibetan Buddhist scholars interpret the two Tibetan syllables of *nang* as inner and *choe* as persuading or motivating change. Therefore, *Nang choe*, or Buddhism, means reasoning that brings about inner evolution.

Nang choe highlights Buddhism's teachings about transforming the mind from suffering and confusion to happiness and enlightenment. This Buddhist philosophy, psychology, and science of the mind are beyond religion. The Four Noble Truths offer an overview of these universal values.

THE FOUR NOBLE TRUTHS

The Buddha taught Four Noble Truths, also called the Middle Way. They are:

1. **The Truth of Suffering**: Life consists of *dukkha*, a Sanskrit term translated as suffering or dis-satisfaction (lack of satisfaction).
2. **The Truth of the Origin of Suffering**: Suffering is caused by ignorance about how to be happy.
3. **The Truth of the Cessation of Suffering**: Liberation from suffering is possible.
4. **The Truth of the Path**: To overcome suffering, live by the Middle Way and Eightfold Path of Ethics.

The Four Noble Truths serve as Tibetan medicine's ethical, spiritual foundation. Through the Four Noble Truths, the Buddha explained steps for cultivating lasting happiness. These guidelines spell out how to evolve and eventually develop an enlightened mind. Because the teachings are profound, they need explanation.

The First Noble Truth

The First Noble Truth states that life consists of suffering. You experience pervasive dissatisfaction for three reasons. First, birth, disease, aging, broken dreams, loss, pain, and death clash with your fantasies about immortality and self-sufficiency. Second, phenomena and experiences that you think lead to happiness, in fact, produce suffering. Third, your conditioning by ignorance, confusion, and bad karma cause you to engage in the three mental poisons.

The First Noble Truth includes the Doctrine of Karma, the process by which ethical behavior leads to happiness and a lack of virtue produces suffering. Karma means "As you sow, so shall you reap" (see chapter 1). When you engage in the three mental poisons, you are out of touch with reality. Alienated from the true nature of mind, you suffer consequently.

According to the Buddha's teachings, your present life is affected by your behavior in your previous existences. Because of unethical behavior and attachment to ego, you have been born again and again in an endless, wearying cycle called *samsara*. Your consciousness goes from one existence to the next one. If the mental poisons pollute your consciousness, this negativity causes suffering in each lifetime.

The First Noble Truth asks you to acknowledge your unethical behavior and resulting suffering. The first step is to recognize the problem. If you don't admit dissatisfaction, you are likely to make excuses for your behavior. You may even try to use distractions to anesthetize your unhappiness, which causes even more suffering.

The Second Noble Truth

The Second Noble Truth states that suffering is caused by fundamental ignorance and confusion about how to be happy. You are attached to your ego, another person, success, honor, ideas, money, and/or material goods. By their very nature, phenomena are impermanent. If you don't accept impermanence, you feel out of control, and you try to make permanent what is only temporary.

You define yourself by your fleeting feelings and attitudes. Because you see everything through the prism of yourself, you crave sensual pleasures. However, they become addictive and perpetuate the dissatisfaction that you want them to alleviate. You spend your precious time and energy defending your ego that doesn't even exist.

The Second Noble Truth recognizes the frustration resulting from the insatiable desire for certainty and permanence. For example, a man was wounded by a bullet. When a physician offered to remove the bullet and treat the wound, the man demanded to know who shot him and what kind of gun was used. He wouldn't let anyone help him until all of his questions were answered. Because he delayed treatment, he died from his injury. Similarly, not acknowledging suffering postpones, perhaps indefinitely, healing and happiness.

The Third Noble Truth

The Third Noble Truth states that liberation from suffering is possible. The world, as interpreted by the senses, is devoid of intrinsic reality. Because all phenomena are in a state of flux, ideas and decisions resulting from the senses lack any real meaning and a solid foundation. Sensory perception is bound to change, stirring up turmoil in the mind. An untamed, unfocused mind indulges in negativity.

The Third Noble Truth explains how to tame the monkey-mind and heal the three mental poisons. Realize the nonexistence of an inherent "self." Then you no longer attribute solidity to phenomena and let fleeting afflictive emotions influence you. Your new understanding changes the way you experience and interpret everything.

The Fourth Noble Truth

The Fourth Noble Truth explains how to free yourself from suffering. Create an enlightened mind. Such a mind is completely awake and not confused by subjectivity. Live by the Middle Way and Eightfold Path of Ethics. Ethics and meditation are the means to transform the mind, allowing it to heal and follow a virtuous path.

As you develop mindfulness, you recognize that your ego is empty of inherent existence. You realize that you couldn't exist without the kindness and support of your parents, friends, teachers, colleagues, and countless other people. Rooting out cravings, you replace them with compassion and wisdom. Turmoil and confusion disappear. You become fully awake.

Finding Refuge

The Four Noble Truths help you to see more clearly and stop taking yourself and others so seriously. You find a safe home—a refuge—in the Buddha, *Dharma*, and *Sangha*. *Sangha* is a Sanskrit word for the community of people who follow Buddhist teachings. Transforming your thinking cultivates peace, goodness, and happiness. Dissatisfaction diminishes. You feel at one with the cosmos and are open to whatever occurs. Your intention is for everyone to be happy and fully awake. You devote your life to helping free all beings from suffering.

THE EIGHTFOLD PATH OF ETHICS

Ethical Behavior

Along with the Four Noble Truths, Buddhism's Eightfold Path of Ethics is the foundation of Tibetan medicine. Behaving ethically protects you from turmoil resulting from unethical behavior. By living according to the Eightfold Path of Ethics, you habituate yourself to virtue. Here is Buddhism's Eightfold Path of Ethics:

1. **Right knowledge**: You come to realize that you are suffering, and the remedy is contained in the Four Noble Truths.
2. **Right aspiration**: You stop behaving in ways that cause suffering for yourself, other people, and the environment; you focus your mind on seeking liberation.
3. **Right speech**: You speak truthfully with compassion.
4. **Right behavior**: You shun violence, practice compassion, and behave responsibly.
5. **Right livelihood**: You do work that promotes ethical behavior and spiritual growth.
6. **Right effort**: You persevere according to the teachings about ethics and spirituality.
7. **Right mindfulness**: You become fully awake and see things as they *really* are.
8. **Right concentration**: You devote your life to ethical living and spiritual practice.

Unethical Behavior

You are more likely to stay the course if you surround yourself with virtuous individuals. Cultivate positive behavior, relationships, and situations. Avoid the ten non-virtuous actions of body, mind, and speech:

1. Killing
2. Stealing
3. Sexual misconduct
4. Lying
5. Divisiveness
6. Harsh speech
7. Senseless speech and gossip
8. Covetousness
9. Harmful intent
10. Wrong view

IMPERMANENCE, EMPTINESS, DEPENDENT ORIGINATION, INTERCONNECTEDNESS

Tibetan Buddhism teaches four profound, interrelated concepts that are essential to Tibetan medicine. These concepts are impermanence, emptiness, dependent origination, and interconnectedness, and they complement each other. They illustrate the absence of an independent self and synergy of everything in the universe. Understanding these concepts will help you create health, happiness, and an enlightened mind.

Impermanence

Impermanence means that all phenomena change continuously. Nothing material is unchanging. Everything and everyone are in a constant state of flux. You and all other living beings are as fleeting as reflections that birds cast when flying over water.

Suffering is not accidental but arises from a specific cause: ignorance. If you are ignorant about impermanence, you misinterpret life and don't realize what will create health and happiness. You suffer by being attached to what is impermanent.

Emptiness

Emptiness in Tibetan Buddhism is complex and misunderstood. Often, emptiness is defined as "empty" or "void," but this definition is inaccurate. Emptiness means that all phenomena are devoid—empty—of inherent existence. Phenomena don't exist alone but are interdependent. Each phenomenon, including you, arises from and is dependent on a complex web of interrelated variables. For example, a wave in the ocean doesn't have a separate existence. A wave is part of and dependent on the ocean.

Emptiness refers to the infinite possibilities of phenomena disappearing, appearing, and changing. For example, the five elements and three *nyepa* constantly shift. They can rise, fall, and/or become disturbed.

That's why creating a healthy mind is essential. Your mind has the potential to heal—and also to destroy. If you don't understand the true nature of mind, you may think that you are separate from everyone and everything. You don't realize that you and all phenomena are part of the energy field. Such confusion fuels egotism and, hence, the three mental poisons.

Dependent Origination

Dependent origination means that all phenomena arise from and are dependent on multiple causes and conditions. Nothing comes into existence or remains in existence by itself. Perceiving a distinct phenomenon is blindness. Everything exists in relation to everything else. Impermanence, emptiness, and dependent origination illustrate synergy and the absence of an independent self.

Because everything consists of energy, a phenomenon can't be separated from its context. You can't be distinguished from the variables that are creating you. The person you are now results from all of your experiences to this point. Your parents, friends, genes, education, work, diet, behavior, and countless other factors influence you.

You suffer if there's a gap between reality and how you view things. When you don't understand dependent origination, you are likely to behave in harmful ways. You interpret everything according to your ego and see yourself as separate from your context. Because of karma, you reap the consequences of this negativity.

A tree, for example, appears to be a distinct object. If you look closely, though, you realize that the tree has no independent existence. In fact, the tree is empty of inherent existence. Rain and snow provide moisture. Wind blows off leaves and branches. Soil and sun nourish the tree. Everything in the universe helps to make the tree what it is. The tree isn't an isolated phenomenon. Because of dependent origination, the tree is dependent on everything else. Of course, you are, too.

Interconnectedness

Interconnectedness means that all phenomena, including you, are made of the same five elements of **earth, water, fire, air,** and **space.** You are born and will die, but the energy field remains. You are part of the energy field, not separate from it. Because all phenomena are interconnected, your every thought, word, and deed—no matter how inconsequential—has implications. Your well-being is intimately connected with the well-being of everyone and everything. It's in your best interest to behave in a manner that avoids suffering and promotes happiness for yourself and everyone else.

Tibetan nomads and yaks illustrate interconnectedness high on the Tibetan plateau. Yaks provide shelter, food, and transportation. The nomad family lives in a yak-skin tent. Inside, a pot simmers over a fire of yak dung and juniper branches. From *dri* (female yak) milk, nomads make cheese, as well as butter to drink in tea and burn in lamps. Yaks are sure-footed on steep, snowy mountain paths. Extreme cold and low oxygen don't bother them. Nomads herd, protect, and feed their yaks. They develop emotional bonds with them, as if they were members of the family.

If you recognize the dreamlike quality of conventional life, you stop trying to make permanent what is impermanent. Your suffering ceases when you realize the interconnectedness of all phenomena. Everyone is in the same boat. Universal compassion results from understanding impermanence, emptiness, dependent origination, and interconnectedness.

UNIVERSAL COMPASSION

Tibetan Spiritual Practices

Tibetans created spiritual practices to cultivate universal compassion, compassion toward everything and everyone, including yourself. When Tibetans converted to Buddhism in the eighth century, they kept some beliefs from *Bon*, Tibet's ancient shamanistic religion. Buddhism and *Bon* became Tibetan Buddhism. Tibetans believe that their practices create *bodhichitta* and an enlightened mind.

Tibetan prayer wheels come from *Bon*. When Tibetans turn prayer wheels, paper scrolls inside send compassion to the world. The turning motion shows that creation and destruction are interconnected: Creation leads to destruction to creation to destruction. This cycle continues indefinitely.

Another *Bon* practice is to string prayer flags over mountain passes, ridges, and rooftops. *Lung-ta*, translated as Wind Horse, is the Tibetan word for prayer flags. They are rectangular cloths in the primary colors representing the five elements from which all phenomena arise. Prayer flags have texts and symbols about Tibetan Buddhist concepts, such as compassion and wisdom. Blowing in the air, prayer flags spread compassion and wisdom around the world.

Still another *Bon* practice is to paint stones white on mountain slopes. Tibetans write on these stones the beloved Sanskrit mantra *Om Mani Padme Hum*, as explained in chapter 5. *Mani* stones represent universal compassion and wisdom.

Tibetans chant *Om Mani Padme Hum* and other mantras to transform negativity into universal compassion and wisdom. Mantra is a Sanskrit word or group of words believed to have spiritual and psychological powers. Systematically chanting a mantra can uncover the true nature of mind and create an enlightened mind.

Tibetan Buddhist nuns and monks carve an image, called a mandala, in colored sand as an expression of universal compassion and wisdom. For example, they may create a Medicine Buddha Mandala for healing. At the end of the mandala ceremony, they sweep up the sand and put it in a river or other flowing body of water to illustrate impermanence and share the blessings with other beings. A mandala, a road map of the universe, depicts the interconnectedness of the universe, human body, and consciousness. The internet has many pictures of a mandala.

When a great lama or spiritual teacher dies, Tibetans search for the next incarnation. Meditation, dreams, and portents help to locate a gifted child who, they believe, is the lama reborn. They groom the child to take over the deceased lama's duties. For centuries, Tibetans have engaged in such practices and still do today to promote universal compassion and wisdom.

Tibetan Buddhist Teachers

Tibetan Buddhist teachers define universal compassion as nonviolence, kindness, and interreligious understanding, even in the face of aggression. To promote universal compassion, they have identified several hundred thousand operations of the mind. They have created meditations to cultivate a clear mind, good heart, and enlightenment.

Tibetan Buddhist teachers travel around the world to give teachings and meet heads of state. They point out the plight of poor, sick, and suffering individuals. Furthermore, they advocate respect for the natural world and healing of the environment. At universities, they call for scholarly work to develop a scientific understanding of the mind.

To promote religious harmony, they hold dialogues with religious leaders, educators, health professionals, scientists, and the public. They recognize that the major wisdom traditions have significant differences, but each one has the potential to create good human beings. Adhering to one wisdom tradition may be helpful on a personal level, they say, but multiple wisdom traditions are necessary for diverse communities. They encourage believers to respect and value each other's practices.

Likewise, the world has many cuisines. Each cuisine can nourish body and mind. With many food options, the world is more interesting and delicious than if only one cuisine existed.

As Tibetan Buddhism moves to the West, so do the teachings about universal compassion. Scientists conduct research about compassion. Religious leaders promote interfaith forums to understand each other's traditions. Health professionals attend workshops about providing compassionate care. Therapists coach clients to practice self-compassion. Teachers educate students about how to behave with compassion.

Cultivating Universal Compassion

Tibetan Buddhism advocates evolving to a high ethical, spiritual level of universal compassion. What is universal compassion in this sense? The understanding that all humans want to be happy and avoid suffering. Universal compassion results from a healthy, disciplined mind and kind, forgiving, peaceful, generous, responsible behavior.

Cultivating universal compassion requires expert guidance. Lack of an ethical, spiritual education can lead to negativity and poor choices. Tibetan medicine recommends learning from compassionate, wise teachers who "walk the talk." Avoid teachers who are poor role models. Study the world's great ethical and spiritual texts.

Cultivating universal compassion means to open your heart to the world's suffering. Reach out to help others, without strings attached. Being openhearted strengthens you, rather than weakens you. You behave with integrity by living up to your best values. Life has meaning because you are making a difference.

As you develop universal compassion, layers of negativity fall away. Your inner wisdom flows spontaneously in all your cells. You come to realize that you are, in fact, happy. Happiness is a lasting, joyful state resulting from a healthy mind. Living ethically and openheartedly is the cause and result of happiness.

By choosing to live in this way, you create an enlightened mind. You evolve into an accomplished ethical, spiritual practitioner and uncover your radiant, fathomless Buddha nature. Mindful of being interconnected with everyone and everything, you are a compassionate, wise, healing presence in the world.

MEDITATION ON THE MEDICINE BUDDHA

Besides behaving ethically, meditating on the Medicine Buddha will help you to cultivate an enlightened mind. The Medicine Buddha is the symbol of Tibetan medicine and an enlightened mind. As chapter 15 describes, research affirms that meditation boosts immunity and promotes a peaceful, focused mind.

Like everyone else, you have the potential to be a Buddha. A Buddha has become liberated from suffering, realized enlightenment, and ended the cycle of birth and death (*samsara*). An "Awakened One" sees the true nature of reality.

The internet has many illustrations of the Buddha. The Buddha's halo, knot on the head, and long earlobes illustrate enlightenment. Dressed in monks' clothes, the Buddha is not attached to material wealth. The Buddha meditates in the lotus position or stands strong and peaceful, regardless of circumstances. The Buddha's body may be painted a primary color: yellow for insight, green for harmony, red for passion, white for purity, and blue for healing. You meditate on the Buddha that represents what you need. For example, meditate on the White Buddha to purify mind and body.

The aquamarine or Blue Buddha is the Medicine Buddha. This Buddha represents healing energy. The Medicine Buddha offers medicine (*Dharma*) to heal suffering. The Medicine Buddha's left hand carries a bowl of healing nectar. The right hand holds a healing plant, *Arura (Terminalia chebula)*.

To do this meditation, visualize yourself as the Medicine Buddha. You can enhance the visualization by chanting the Medicine Buddha Mantra or listening to someone else chant the mantra. The internet has pictures of the Medicine Buddha, as well as audiotapes and videotapes of Tibetans chanting the Medicine Buddha Mantra. By listening carefully, you will learn how to pronounce this shortened version of the Medicine Buddha Mantra:

> *Ta dya tha*
> *Om beishajye beishajye*
> *Maha beishajye beishajye*
> *Raja samung gate svaha.*

Tibetan medicine practitioners ascribe great efficacy to the Medicine Buddha Meditation. Before doing a consultation and administering Tibetan medicines and other therapies, they visualize themselves as the Medicine Buddha and chant the Medicine Buddha Mantra. They believe that the meditation transforms them into true healers and makes the treatment more potent. At someone's deathbed, they do the Medicine Buddha Meditation to help the individual transition peacefully to the next sphere of existence.

When you wake up in the morning, do the Medicine Buddha Meditation to be a healing presence throughout the day. Visualize yourself as the Medicine Buddha if you are upset, getting sick, or are ill and need healing. At someone's sickbed or deathbed, do the meditation to be a true healer. On your deathbed, visualizing yourself as the Medicine Buddha will heal your mind, even though your body is dying.

While cultivating a healthy, enlightened mind, you also need to meet your daily physical needs. Otherwise, your three primary energies will go out of balance, and you will experience suffering and pain that monopolize your attention. You will have little time and energy left to live happily and do acts of loving-kindness. The next chapter explains how to create a healthy body. You can adapt the guidelines to your unique constitution and health status.

· 8 ·

Create a Healthy Body

*T*ibetan medicine teaches that suffering begins in the mind. ***Loong,*** ***tripa,*** and ***baekan,*** the three primary energies or *nyepa,* are essential for life. Under the influence of the three mental poisons, however, the *nyepa* are the source of suffering. Greed, attachment, and desire, the first mental poison, cause and result from ***loong*** energy. Anger, hostility, and aggression, the second mental poison, produce and result from ***tripa*** energy. Delusion, confusion, and closed-mindedness, the third mental poison, give rise to and result from ***baekan*** energy.

You undermine yourself by engaging in the three mental poisons. This mind-set leads to poor choices and dysfunction. Your *nyepa* rise too high, fall too low, and/or become disturbed. If the current percentages of your *nyepa* are out of sync with your constitution, your organs, passages, channels, and cells overflow, become blocked, are diverted, and/or get disturbed. To create a healthy body, you need to create a healthy mind and make choices that help you to live in harmony with your constitution.

You learn about your unique strengths and vulnerabilities by doing a systematic analysis of your constitution, as described in chapter 2. Knowing who you *really* are helps you to make informed choices to keep your *nyepa* in balance. Proactive steps support your body to function well and avoid conditions leading to suffering and disease.

This chapter explains how to create a healthy body by making good choices about your diet, digestion, and behavior. You learn to adjust to daily, seasonal, and environmental changes and to rejuvenate yourself. If you create a personalized plan, you can adapt the recommendations to your own unique constitution and health status. Your

129

plan won't be a quick fix, especially if your *nyepa* are out of balance. By making changes slowly, you will identify which ones help you to be healthier and happier. The chapter ends with Tibetan Prostrations, an ancient meditation to purify mind and body.

DIET

Support Your Constitution

You maximize your health and longevity by ingesting a diet that supports your unique constitution. Everything in the universe is comprised of the five sources of energy, or elements: **earth**, **water**, **fire**, **air**, and **space**. Thus, everything is potential medicine or poison. To create a healthy body, you need to make informed choices about what to eat and drink. Ingest what keeps the current percentages of your *nyepa* about the same as their percentages in your constitution.

Select a variety of wholesome foods and beverages that ideally are organic, fresh, unpolluted, natural, and grown locally. Develop mindfulness about how foods and beverages affect you. Learn which ones produce appropriate grounding, heating, cooling, and energy. Avoid those that lead to indigestion, imbalance, and lack of energy.

For example, potatoes and other vegetables that grow in the ground generally have a cooling effect on gastritis and nausea. If you have a *baekan* constitution, however, potatoes may not be good for you because they increase the **earth** and **water** elements. Peanuts can be excellent for you, especially in winter. They increase heat in the body and pacify *loong* disorders. Even so, peanuts are contraindicated if you have a *tripa* constitution, high cholesterol, elevated blood pressure, and heart ailments, or you are allergic to peanuts.

Make Healthy Choices about Fruits and Vegetables

Choose fruits and vegetables that keep your *nyepa* in sync with your constitution. Fruits and vegetables have different potencies depending on their makeup of the five elements. Some heat you up and others cool you down.

For example, *baekan* increases in winter cold, which can decrease *tripa*. To reverse this imbalance, eat warm, spicy vegetables to warm *baekan* and increase *tripa*. Summer heat causes *tripa* to rise and *baekan* to fall. Fresh salads and other cooling fruits and vegetables cool *tripa* and increase *baekan*.

How Plants Affect **Loong**, **Tripa**, *and* **Baekan**

- Plants with the quality of **earth**, such as potatoes, grow in the ground or away from the sun; they aggravate *baekan* and pacify *loong*.
- Plants with the quality of **water**, such as zucchini and potatoes, aggravate *baekan* and pacify *tripa*.
- Plants with the quality of **fire**, such as hot peppers, grow in the sun; they aggravate *tripa* and pacify *baekan*.
- Plants with the quality of **air**, such as lettuce, aggravate *loong* and pacify *baekan*.

Learn about how fruits and vegetables affect you. Be mindful of their taste and how you feel after eating them. Fruits like lemons and limes are sour and produce heat. Bananas and other sweet fruits increase *baekan* and can lead to weight gain.

Some vegetables taste hot or pungent on the tongue, whereas others are sour. Vegetables taste bitter if collected from cold, dry locations and used in dried or cooked forms. Bitter vegetables, such as bitter gourd, are light and cooling in quality and reduce hot imbalance. Vegetables from hot or tropical regions are warm in quality and decrease cold disorders.

Make Healthy Choices about Seeds and Grains

Sesame seeds, which are heavy and warm in quality, pacify *loong*. Linseeds, with a sweet, bitter taste and oily, smooth qualities, treat *loong* disorders. Buckwheat, being cool and light in quality, improves blood circulation and heals wounds but also aggravates all three *nyepa*. The taste and post-digestive tastes of wheat, barley, and rice are sweet, which pacify *loong* and increase *baekan*. Wheat, which is heavy and cool, pacifies *loong* and *tripa*. Barley's heavy, cool quality regulates bowel movements and promotes overall well-being. However, roasted barley, which Tibetans use to make *tsampa*, becomes light in nature and improves ***tripa***-related indigestion, such as acid reflux and heartburn.

Cooked white rice treats diarrhea and vomiting as well as corrects imbalances in the *nyepa*. If cooked in water, rice is light and easily digested. Rice boiled in consommé or milk is heavy in quality. Cooked rice porridge with a light consistency quenches thirst, is refreshing, treats gastroenteritis, enhances digestion, balances the body constituents, generates digestive heat, and makes the channels flexible. Cooked rice porridge having a medium consistency generates body heat, satiates hunger, quenches thirst, treats weakness and lethargy, stimulates digestion, and eases constipation. Cooked rice porridge with a heavy consistency quenches thirst but can lead to weight gain.

Make Healthy Choices about Legumes

Beans taste sweet and astringent. Cool and light in quality, they block the openings of the channels, reduce hot disorders associated with ***baekan***, treat diarrhea, and dissolve fats. Broad beans, or fava beans, relieve combined disorders of ***baekan*** and ***loong***. They treat asthma and hemorrhoids but worsen blood and ***tripa*** disorders. Lentils taste sweet and astringent, which aggravates all three *nyepa*. When used in a paste form, lentils treat gout and blood disorders. Kidney beans pacify ***loong*** disorders and increase ***baekan***, ***tripa***, and sperm counts.

Make Healthy Choices about Meat

Treat all beings kindly. Killing for sport is unethical. Like human beings, animals, birds, and fish are sentient because they have the capacity to feel, perceive, and experience. Killing them is justifiable only if eating them is essential for health. When your health requires eating animals, birds, and fish as food, kill them in an ethical manner that avoids suffering.

If you choose to eat animals, only ingest small portions of organic, clean, free-range, lean, cooked, and easily digested meat. Individuals with ***loong*** disorders may benefit from eating meat. Broth made with meat and/or bones promotes physical strength and satiates hunger.

Beef and chicken, being warm in quality, aggravate *tripa* and pacify *loong* and *baekan*. Buffalo meat is warming, induces sleep, and increases weight. Mutton and lamb, which are oily and warm in quality, increase energy, develop body constituents, pacify *loong* and *baekan* disorders, and improve appetite. Yak meat, which is oily and warm in quality, increases *tripa* and treats disorders associated with *baekan*. Rabbit meat, rough in quality, generates heat and decreases diarrhea. Eating fish heals stomach disorders, improves appetite, clears eyesight, treats cancer, and warms *baekan*.

Not all meats are warming. Goat meat is cool and light in quality and pacifies *tripa*. Pork, though cooling, can increase *tripa* due to its dense fat content.

Eat the Six Tastes Each Day

The five elements consist of six tastes: sweet, sour, salty, bitter, pungent, and astringent. All six tastes are needed to create and maintain health. Choosing a diet with the six tastes replenishes the five elements and keeps the three *nyepa* in balance.

Six Tastes and Foods to Ingest for Each Taste

Sweet   The sweet taste clings to the mouth and causes craving for more. Composed of **earth** and **water** elements, the sweet taste is heavy, moist, and cooling. Sweet decreases *loong* and *tripa* and increases *baekan*. These foods contain the sweet taste:

- Most grains such as wheat, rice, barley, and corn.
- Maple syrup, milk, and milk products such as butter, *ghee* (clarified butter), and cream.
- Fruits such as coconut, date, fig, grape, pear, mango, dried fruit, and banana.
- Vegetables such as potato, sweet potato, carrots, and beet roots.
- Sugar in any form: raw, refined, brown, white, molasses, sugar cane, and honey.

Sour   The sour taste puts the teeth on edge, puckers the face, and makes the mouth water. Composed of **fire** and **earth** elements, sour is hot, light, and moist. Sour decreases *loong* and **baekan**, and increases **tripa**. These foods have a sour taste:

- Fruits such as lemon, lime, orange, pineapple, passion fruit, cherry, and plum.
- Dairy products such as yogurt, cheese, and sour cream.
- Fermented products such as vinegar, pickles, sauerkraut, soy sauce, kimchi, and wine.

Salty   The salty taste creates a hot feeling and increases saliva. Composed of **water** and **fire** elements, salt is hot, heavy, and moist by nature. Salt decreases *loong* and increases *tripa* and **baekan**. These foods have a salty taste:

- Any kind of salt, including rock salt and sea salt.
- Any food or beverage to which salt has been added such as pickles, nuts, and chips.
- Sea vegetables such as seaweed and kelp.

Bitter   The bitter taste may be unpleasant, sharp, and disagreeable. Composed of **water** and **air** elements, bitter is light, cooling, and dry by nature. The bitter taste increases *loong* and decreases *tripa* and *baekan*. These foods have a bitter taste:

- Green leafy vegetables such as dandelion greens, spinach, and kale.
- Zucchini, bitter gourd, and eggplant.
- Herbs and spices such as turmeric and dandelion root.
- Fruits such as citrus peel, grapefruit, and olives.
- Coffee, unsweetened cocoa, and some alcoholic beverages.

Pungent   The pungent taste burns the mouth and tongue and causes the eyes to water. Composed of **fire** and **air** elements, the pungent taste is hot, dry, and light. The pungent taste raises *loong* and *tripa* and lowers *baekan*. These foods have a pungent taste:

- Hot spices such as chili peppers, black pepper, cayenne, mustard seeds, ginger, cumin, cloves, cardamom, garlic, and onions.
- Mild spices such as anise and cinnamon.
- Fresh herbs such as oregano, thyme, and mint.

Astringent The astringent taste sticks to the tongue and palate, creating a rough, sharp feeling. Composed of **earth** and **air** elements, the astringent taste is dry, cooling, and heavy by nature. The astringent taste increases *loong* and *baekan* and decreases *tripa*. These foods have an astringent taste:

- Legumes such as beans and lentils.
- Fruits such as cranberries, pomegranates, pears, banana peel, dried fruit, and most unripe fruit.
- Vegetables such as broccoli, cauliflower, asparagus, turnip, and raw vegetables.
- Grains such as rye, buckwheat, and quinoa.
- Herbs and spices including turmeric, marjoram, cloves, and cinnamon.
- Coffee, tea, red wine, dark chocolate, and vanilla.

Make Healthy Choices about Herbs and Spices

Herbs and spices add taste, nutrition, and attractiveness to food and beverages. They affect mind and body. Ingest herbs and spices that help you to create balance.

How Herbs and Spices Affect Mind and Body

- **Basil**: Purifies and uplifts the heart and mind, decreases excess *baekan* in the lungs, and removes excess *loong* from the colon.
- **Cardamom**: Stimulates digestion and kidney function, as well as helps to balance the heavy, clogging influence of milk.
- **Cinnamon**: Promotes digestion and assists other spices to be absorbed.
- **Cloves**: Decreases excess *loong* and *baekan* but can increase *tripa*.
- **Coriander**: Has a cooling influence, promotes digestion by kindling agni (digestive fire) without aggravating *tripa*, and helps to build up all tissues.
- **Cumin**: Strengthens digestion and metabolizes impurities without aggravating *tripa*.

- **Fennel**: Aids digestion by kindling *agni* without aggravating *tripa* and strengthens the downward flow of elimination.
- **Ginger**: Improves digestion, increases heat, and metabolizes impurities.
- **Mustard**: Stimulates digestion, helps metabolize impurities, and increases *tripa*.
- **Nutmeg** or **Mace**: Calms *loong* and, if consumed in warm milk, enhances sleep.
- **Saffron**: Promotes tissue development and nourishes the whole body.
- **Salt**: Generates heat, enhances digestion, and regulates bowel movements.
- **Turmeric**: Serves as an astringent and antioxidant, purifies tissues, decreases mucus from excess *baekan*, and is recommended for the daily diet.

Make Healthy Choices about Fats

Healthy fats have subtle, sweet, moist qualities. They pacify *loong*, cleanse and lubricate the abdomen and joints, boost body heat, promote physical strength, and create a rosy complexion. Eating fats soothes mental unrest.

After cleansing therapies, eat fat for lubrication. Fats help to heal internal disorders and synthesize body constituents. They strengthen sensory organs and slow aging. However, eating too many and/or unhealthy fats aggravates *baekan* and leads to obesity and related problems.

Butter, seed oils, and animal fat are successively heavier and cooler in quality. Fresh butter is cool in quality and reduces hot disorders associated with *tripa*. Clarified butter (*ghee*) is supreme among fats. *Ghee* sharpens intelligence, enhances memory, generates heat, increases physical strength, and prolongs life. Even so, excessive intake of fats can cause health problems.

Sesame oil, which is hot and sharp in quality, helps to increase weight for underweight individuals, reduce weight for obese persons, firm the body, and relieve combined disorders of *baekan* and *loong*. Mustard oil pacifies *loong* but aggravates *baekan* and *tripa*. Animal fats promote healing of the ear, brain, and uterus.

Make Healthy Choices about Dairy Products

Milk treats the *nyepa* serially (*loong, tripa, baekan*) but aggravates the *nyepa* in reverse order (*baekan, tripa, loong*). The taste and post-digestive tastes of milk are sweet. Milk, having heavy and oily qualities, helps to develop body constituents, improves the complexion, and pacifies combined disorders of *loong* and *tripa*.

Cheese improves the appetite, hardens the stool, and relieves *baekan* disorders. Curd, the soft, white substance formed when milk sours, is used to make cheese. The tastes and post-digestive tastes of all curds are sour. Curd is cool and oily in quality, eases hard stools, pacifies *loong*, and stimulates appetite. Curd water cleanses the channels and causes loose bowel movements. Whey, the liquid remaining after milk has been curdled and strained, treats *baekan* problems without aggravating *loong* and *tripa*.

Make Healthy Choices about Water

Pure, boiled water, cooled enough to drink, is THE primordial, essential medicine. This ideal beverage helps to increase digestive heat and pacify *baekan*. Drinking pure, boiled water breaks down fats, reduces toxins, and relieves hiccups. Moreover, this beverage treats indigestion, stomach distention, abdominal cramps, asthma, and the common cold.

Drink pure, boiled, cooled water before meals, during meals, or after meals to lose weight, maintain weight, and gain weight, respectively. After meals, drink this ideal beverage to spread the nutrients throughout your body and increase your strength. Regularly drinking this beverage will help to keep your *nyepa* in balance.

Pure, boiled water that is cooled enough to drink treats *tripa* disorders. Examples are fainting, fatigue, vomiting, hangovers, dizziness, thirst, and poisoning. In contrast, ice water lowers digestive heat and slows digestion, which can produce toxins from undigested food. Icy beverages can be harmful for people with a *loong* and/or *baekan* constitution.

Avoid drinking impure water, such as standing water and water contaminated with chemicals, preservatives, plastics, and other toxins. Don't drink water that has microorganisms, dirt, insects, droppings, algae, grass, leaves, and other pollutants. Boiled water can become toxic if left in the open too long. Ocean water is too salty for the body.

Make Healthy Choices about Alcohol

Generally, alcohol has a sweet, sour, bitter taste and a sour post-digestive taste. Alcohol generates heat, gives rise to courage, induces sleep, and relieves combined disorders of **baekan** and **loong**. Drinking a small amount of alcohol with or after meals can increase digestive heat if you have a **loong** and/or **baekan** constitution. A small amount of alcohol can help you gain weight if you have a **loong** constitution.

However, alcohol can cause mild diarrhea because of its sharp, warm, rough, subtle quality. Alcohol is contraindicated if you are overweight. Excessive intake of alcohol produces mental unrest, abnormal behavior, indiscretion, lack of responsibility, and shamelessness. Avoid alcohol if you have a **tripa** constitution. Alcohol increases **tripa** and promotes heat-related disorders. If you have a **loong** and/or **tripa** constitution, you are prone to developing alcoholism.

Avoid Harmful Foods

Safeguard your health by avoiding what aggravates your *nyepa*. A beverage or food that changes in color, smell, and/or taste may not be safe. Stale food destroys digestive heat, lacks nutrition, and produces toxins. If you are allergic to something, avoid it. Don't drink or eat what causes sleep disturbance, indigestion, headaches, mental unrest, skin rashes, and other distress.

Stay away from foods and beverages that generally are incompatible and can become toxic. However, you may not be adversely affected if you are used to eating them, you have a **tripa** constitution, and you are healthy with strong digestive heat. Otherwise, you are best off steering clear of them and other foods and beverages that can poison you. For example, a cheeseburger, french fries, and iced soda can make you sick.

Food Combinations That Can Be Toxic

- Alcohol with curd before it is set
- Fish with milk
- Milk with some fruits
- Fish with chicken eggs
- Mushrooms fried in mustard oil
- Chicken with curd

- Honey with an equal amount of oil from grains
- Fresh butter preserved in a metal vessel for a length of time
- Iced drinks with foods that are hard to digest, such as green salads, or contain fat, such as salad dressings (cold solidifies fat, making it difficult to digest)
- Cooked food kept in an unrefrigerated airtight container
- Milk with sour food
- Any food before the previous meal is digested

You may enjoy sampling foods and beverages that aren't in your usual diet, especially when you travel in a foreign country. If so, don't suddenly change your diet, or you may get sick. Gradually add to your diet safe, nutritious, unfamiliar foods and beverages. Slowly decrease what you ordinarily eat and drink. In a nutshell, eat moderate portions of what nourishes you and doesn't harm you.

DIGESTION

Support Strong Digestive Heat

Strong digestive heat is crucial to support the *nyepa*, the seven body constituents (nutritional essence, blood, muscular tissue, fat, bone, bone marrow, regenerative fluid), and the three waste products (feces, urine, sweat). Given proper digestive heat, the body digests food particles, without creating toxins, and sustains the body constituents. As a result, waste products move downward for normal defecation and urination.

Strong digestive heat promotes physical strength, a healthy complexion, and longevity. Digestive *tripa* is the primary energy in digestive heat. Healthy action of digestive heat enables the body to complete all eight steps of successful digestion.

Healthy Digestive Heat Produces These Actions

1. Food is swallowed and moves through the esophagus toward the stomach with help from life-sustaining *loong*.
2. Liquid softens the food for further digestion.
3. Fire-accompanying *loong* helps digestive *tripa* to increase heat.

4. Digestion in the stomach resembles the boiling of medicinal ingredients in a pot.
5. Decomposing **baekan** breaks down the food and transforms it into a sweet, bubbly substance that generates more **baekan** energy.
6. Digestive **tripa** further digests and heats the food, transforming it into a sour substance called *chyle*, which generates more **tripa** energy.
7. Fire-accompanying **loong** separates *chyle* into nutritional essence and waste.
8. Nutritional essence, with its bitter taste, generates more **loong** and nourishes the body.

Poor digestive heat is a major cause of imbalance. If food is not digested properly, undigested food particles move through the digestive system, create toxins, and harm the body constituents. To strengthen digestive heat, ingest a warm diet that supports your constitution. Avoid cold foods and beverages that reduce your digestive heat.

If your constitution is **loong**, your digestive heat most likely is unstable, and you have hard stools, especially when you travel and aren't grounded. Ordinarily, a **tripa** constitution produces strong digestive heat and loose stools. Typically, a **baekan** constitution creates weak digestive heat and stools that are medium in consistency. In a dual constitution, digestive heat and stools reflect both dominant energies.

Eat and Drink Appropriately

A healthy body requires dietary practices that promote immediate, easy digestion. Appropriate eating and drinking habits generate strong digestive heat and sustain life. For optimal digestion, engage in healthy dietary practices.

Healthy Dietary Practices

- Make healthy food choices.
- Only eat and drink what you need to nourish your body.
- Eat according to your hunger level: Only eat when you are hungry and avoid eating when you are not hungry.

- Eat at approximately the same times every day.
- Eat and drink sitting in a relaxed environment, not too quickly or too slowly.
- Express gratefulness for each plant and sentient being that gives its life for you.
- Chew your food well; digestion begins in the mouth.
- Fill your stomach one-half with solid food, one-fourth with water, and one-fourth empty to accommodate *loong*.
- Allow three to six hours between meals or undigested food may mix with partially digested food and cause indigestion.

Inadequate, excessive, or adverse intake can cause disease and even death. Undereating promotes *loong* disorders. Excessive eating cools *tripa*, aggravates *baekan*, and leads to indigestion and obesity. Overeating gives rise to too much mucus that blocks the channels of fire-accompanying *loong* and decreases digestive heat. Adverse eating, such as ingesting harmful foods and beverages, causes imbalance in all three *nyepa* and produces complicated illnesses that are challenging to unravel.

You can determine the correct amount of foods to eat by their quantity, the size of your stomach, and the strength of your digestive heat. Appropriate intake creates a healthy body and proper functioning of the *nyepa*. When you consistently follow healthy dietary practices for your unique constitution, your appetite is good, your digestive heat is strong, and you develop physical strength. Good digestion clears the sensory organs, lightens the body, and eases the elimination of feces, flatus, and urine.

BEHAVIOR

Avoid Getting Sick

To create a healthy body, train yourself to behave in a manner that promotes your health and long life. Avoid stale, polluted air that brings toxins into your body, depletes your energy, and causes disease. Breathe properly to fill your lungs with fresh, clean air. Engaging in circular breathing helps to get rid of toxins and oxygenate each cell. Circular breathing is part of each meditation in this book: Breathe through your nose, from your abdomen, slowly deeply and evenly, with your in-breath the same length as your out-breath, and no break in between.

Summon up your courage to avoid getting sick. Promptly notice when your *nyepa* are out of balance and bring them back into harmony again. Try not to overuse, underuse, and misuse your body, mind, or speech. Protect yourself from communicable diseases. Visualize being a Medicine Buddha who heals all suffering and illness.

Sleep Well

Sleep comfortably and deeply for as long as you need. Wake up refreshed in the morning. Without sufficient sleep, you will depress your immune system. Moreover, you will lose your physical and mental strength and develop a *loong* disorder.

Before going to bed, take steps to sleep well. Here are some suggestions to help you sleep: Sip warm broth or warm milk with nutmeg. Eat some cottage cheese or another food with calcium. Apply oil on the crown of your head and behind your ears. A regular oil massage, especially on your head, feet, and ears, can help you to sleep through the night.

Daytime sleep and too much sleep aggravate **baekan** and cause swelling, headaches, lethargy, and obesity. Avoid sleeping during the day unless you are weak, tired, and/or sick. If you are intoxicated, you may need to sleep during the day. A nap may be beneficial if your *loong* is high and you are anxious, stressed-out, or depressed. Napping replenishes elders. You may need a nap if you don't get enough sleep at night.

Be Responsible about Sexual Activity

Behave according to ethical values and norms involving sexual activity. Avoid hurting yourself or anyone else. Cultivate openness, honesty, compassion, and nonviolence in relationships. Be moderate in sexual activity. Excessive sex for your constitution and stage in life will deplete your **loong** and **tripa** and cause you to die prematurely.

Exercise Appropriately

Moderation is needed regarding physical exercise, too. Proper exercise produces lightness of the body and a good figure. Appropriate exercise burns toxins and improves muscle tone. Toning the body promotes efficiency in doing daily activities. Suitable exercise increases metabolism and digestive heat, as well as reduces indigestion.

However, too much exercise is harmful, especially for children and elders. If you have a *loong* and/or *tripa* constitution, you are best off exercising moderately, or your *loong* and *tripa* may rise too high and produce *loong* and *tripa* disorders. Eventually, your *loong* and *tripa* will become depleted, giving rise to complex diseases that involve all three *nyepa*. If your constitution is *baekan*, you need to exercise regularly and vigorously, or your *baekan* will increase and you will feel sluggish and gain weight.

Practice Cleanliness and Orderliness

Live and work in clean, toxin-free environments with fresh, pure air. Cleanliness decreases lethargy, generates digestive heat, shuns illness, and prolongs life. Wash your body each day. You will decrease rashes, perspiration, elevated body heat, and foul body odor. To promote the free flow of energy, keep your home, workplace, and life organized and uncluttered.

DAILY, SEASONAL, AND ENVIRONMENTAL CHANGES

Adjust to Daily Changes

When the three primary energies—*loong, tripa,* and *baekan*—function well, they rise and fall every twelve hours. You are best off adapting to their natural cycle. Set up a healthy, daily routine that is consistent with the rise and fall of your *nyepa*.

Healthy, Daily Routine Consistent with the Rise and Fall of the Nyepa

- **3–7 a.m. *Loong* active**: You have a tendency for mental alertness. Get up before 7 a.m. when *baekan* begins rising. Evacuate your bowel and bladder. Clean your teeth, tongue, and sinuses. Wash your body. Dress in clean, comfortable, natural fabrics.

Do breathing techniques and exercise to increase your metabolism and oxygenate your tissues. Meditate.

- **7-11 a.m.** *Baekan* **active**: You have a tendency for physical heaviness, mental slowness, and feeling cold. Eat a light, warm breakfast because your digestive heat is low. Avoid sleeping. Exercise. Work.
- **11 a.m. to 3 p.m.** *Tripa* **active**: Your tendency is to be warm. Work in a cool area. Eat your main meal around noon when digestive heat is strong. Relax for about ten minutes after eating.
- **3–7 p.m.** *Loong* **active**: Your tendency is to be tired. Work. Exercise. Eat a light evening meal by 6:30 p.m. Because your digestion is slow, avoid heavy, cold foods and beverages that produce indigestion and toxins. Rest for about ten minutes after eating.
- **7-11 p.m.** *Baekan* **active**: You have a tendency for physical heaviness and mental slowness. Relax. Take a walk or do gentle yoga postures. Listen to calming music or read a book you enjoy. Go to bed by 10:30 p.m. and be sound asleep by 11 p.m. when *tripa* starts rising.
- **11 p.m. to 3 a.m.** *Tripa* **active**: Your tendency is to be warm. Sleep soundly to burn off toxins. Without nightly metabolic housekeeping, toxins will increase, giving rise to imbalance and disease.

Acclimate to Seasonal Changes

Depending on where you live, the weather may vary greatly from winter, to spring, to summer, and to fall. These change exert a big effect on mind and body. You need to adjust your environment, clothes, and behavior to the season. Moreover, ingest tastes and qualities of foods according to the season. Table 8.1 explains how to adjust your diet to seasonal changes.

In winter, cold temperatures and *loong* cause body pores to close and *baekan* to accumulate. You feel sluggish and physically weak if you aren't warm enough, especially in the lower part of your torso. A sesame oil massage, vigorous exercise, and a warm diet will heat you up. Wear warm clothes and shoes. Keep your home and workplace at a comfortable temperature.

Table 8.1. **Adjust Your Diet to Seasonal Changes**

Season	Tastes to Consume	Qualities to Consume
Winter	Sweet, Sour, Salty	Warm
Spring	Bitter, Hot, Astringent	Rough
Summer	Sweet	Cool
Fall	Sweet, Sour, Salty	Warm

During a cold, wet spring, *baekan* may increase, causing digestive heat to decrease. You are susceptible to developing a *baekan* disorder, such as the common cold. Exercise regularly to raise your metabolism. Relax in the sun on a warm day.

Hot weather in summer increases *tripa* and depletes physical strength. Avoid vigorous exercise and stay out of the hot sun. Take cool showers or baths. Ingest a cooling diet. Wear thin, light clothes. Keep your home and workplace cool and well ventilated. Relax under a shady tree in a light breeze.

Rain, wind, and cool temperatures in the fall increase *baekan* and depress digestive heat. Engage in behavior that generates digestive heat. Examples are exercising vigorously, increasing your metabolism, and eating spicy food. Keep your home and workplace warm and dry. Avoid damp, cold places.

Adapt to Environmental Changes

If you travel, you may find that the altitude, climate, food, people, and culture are different from what you are used to. You need to adapt to these changes. Tibetans are an example of why adjusting to a different environment is essential for health.

The Tibetan plateau averages three miles high. The high altitude and cold, dry climate are not favorable for growing fruits and vegetables. Traditionally, Tibetans ate *tsampa (roasted barley flour)* and yak meat, butter, and cheese. They drank black tea with salt and yak milk and butter. This diet kept them lubricated, nourished, and warm. Tibetans who leave their homeland for sea-level locations must adjust to the lower altitude and warmer, often moister weather. Ingesting the same diet as in Tibet makes them prone to diabetes, hypertension, obesity, and other health problems.

REJUVENATION

As you age, your body constituents and physical strength gradually diminish. You will develop health problems and shorten your life span unless you take steps to slow the aging process. By rejuvenating yourself regularly, you can prolong your youthful appearance, boost your energy, and extend your life. You will benefit from daily, monthly, and yearly rejuvenation.

Rejuvenate yourself in a place that is clean, quiet, pleasant, and free of disturbance. Clean yourself inside and out to get rid of toxins in your body, mind, and life. Take time to relax, heal, and restore your body and mind.

For advice about rejuvenation, you can consult with a qualified, experienced Tibetan medicine practitioner. The practitioner will analyze your constitution, *nyepa*, and internal organs. Then the practitioner will prescribe a rejuvenation protocol for you.

To prepare for rejuvenation, the practitioner may recommend a steam bath, oil massage, cleansing bath, and/or shower. In addition, the practitioner may prescribe Tibetan medicines to remove toxins. After your body is clean inside and out, the practitioner will administer the rejuvenation protocol.

You can rejuvenate yourself by meditating and walking safely in nature. Periodically stop your daily activities and focus on your breath for two minutes. Extend these short meditations to longer periods of time. Doing Tibetan Prostrations each day will revitalize your mind and body.

MEDITATION: TIBETAN PROSTRATIONS

Tibetans do prostrations to meditate, show respect, decrease ego, and develop good karma (positive energy). At Tibetan Buddhist sacred sites, Tibetans do at least three prostrations in front of the Buddha statute and/or high lama. Some Tibetans do thousands of prostrations to burn off bad karma (negative energy), often putting carpet pieces on their hands and knees to protect them. Yoga Sun Salutations, a sequence of yoga poses, may be based on the ancient meditation practice of Tibetan Prostrations.

Tibetan Prostrations help to tone the body, release nervous energy, and focus the mind. They calm and harmonize body and mind. The internet has videos showing Tibetans performing Tibetan Prostrations.

How to Meditate while Doing Tibetan Prostrations

- Stand tall and sturdy in Mountain, a yoga pose called *Tadasana* in Sanskrit, with your feet pointing straight ahead and about hip-width apart.
- Keep your spine tall and relaxed, arms hanging at your sides with your palms turned inward toward your hips, and toes stretched out.
- Align the middle of your ear, your shoulder, and the sides of your hip, knee, and ankle along an imaginary vertical line.
- Place your palms together (Prayer Pose) at your Heart Chakra, smile slightly, and relax your eyes.
- Lower your eyes, without bending your head, and look at the ground or floor a short distance in front of you.
- Engage in circular breathing: Breathe through your nose, from your abdomen, slowly deeply and evenly, with your in-breath the same length as your out-breath, and no break in between; continue circular breathing during and after the prostrations.
- Place your hands in Prayer Pose at your Crown Chakra, then at your Brow Chakra, then at your Throat Chakra, and then back to your Heart Chakra.
- Kneel, put your hands flat under your shoulders, and touch your forehead to the ground or floor; for a full-length prostration, push your hands out in front of you and lie flat with your forehead touching the ground or floor.
- Stand up in Mountain Pose, with your hands in Prayer Pose at your Heart Chakra.
- Do at least three Tibetan Prostrations.
- Stand up in Mountain Pose, with your hands in Prayer Pose at your Heart Chakra and let your heart rate, breathing, and blood pressure return to normal.
- Open your eyes and continue to engage in circular breathing.

In summary, you can improve the health of your body by making good choices about diet, digestion, and behavior. Adjust to daily, seasonal, and environmental changes, and rejuvenate yourself regularly. Do Tibetan Prostrations to help you to settle down, strengthen yourself, and harmonize mind and body.

No matter how healthy your mind and body are, though, you eventually will die. Some wisdom traditions teach two perspectives on what occurs after death: (1) You go to heaven or hell, depending on how you lived your life, or (2) you cease to exist. Tibetan medicine teaches a third perspective: Your consciousness will transition from life, to death, to an intermediate state called the bardo, to rebirth.

· 9 ·

Create a Good Death

$\mathcal{T}$ibetan Buddhism, the foundation of Tibetan medicine, doesn't advocate belief in an anthropomorphic, interventionist god. God is all the conscious energy infusing everyone and everything in the universe. Conscious energy is the very source of existence. You, like all living beings, are a manifestation of this life force, just as a wave is part of the ocean. A god doesn't reward you with happiness or punish you with suffering. Because of karma, you create your own happiness and suffering, depending on your choices. Karma means "as you sow, so shall you reap," as explained in chapter 1.

You die like you live. Therefore, the art of dying is as important as the art of living. The quality of your dying process and next rebirth results from karma you created in your previous lives and in this life. When your body dies, your life doesn't end. You are reborn. *Samsara* is the Sanskrit term for the cycle of life, death, intermediate state, and rebirth. In each stage, you develop a corresponding change in consciousness.

The Tibetan word bardo means a gap or transition between one situation and another one. Most often, bardo refers to the intermediate state between death and rebirth. You cycle through *samsara* until you purify your bad karma (negative energy) and create an enlightened mind. Through ethical behavior and meditation, you can come to understand and experience these stages with peace and even joy, rather than fear.

This chapter explains how to create harmonious transitions through life, death, the bardo, and rebirth. These teachings are comforting, even if you don't believe in rebirth. You can use the teachings to provide compassionate care for persons who are dying, including

149

yourself. The chapter ends with steps for doing Tonglen Meditation while you or someone else is dying.

LIFE

Prepare for Death

Tibet's ancient science of healing, commonly known as Tibetan medicine, advocates creating a long, healthy, happy life. In addition to meeting your own needs, you reach out to help others and heal the world. Living in this way produces meaning, seeing your life as part of a bigger purposeful picture. You behave with integrity by rising to your best self. When your body and mind are worn out, you let go and die, rather than prolong suffering needlessly.

You can't escape death. No matter what quality of life you create, you will die. Although death is certain, the time, place, and manner of death are uncertain. You may die at any time, in any circumstance, and at any place. A single breath, or when consciousness separates from the body, is all that distinguishes life and death. That's why fear of death underlies all other fears. Transforming this fear into a peaceful, compassionate mind is essential to live and die well.

Creating a peaceful, compassionate mind during life gives rise to a peaceful dying process. After you meet your basic needs, accumulating possessions and accomplishments won't help you to die well. To die peacefully, you must let go of your attachments to possessions, success, family, and friends. Unless you train yourself to let go during life, you will have difficulty letting go when your body and mind are worn out and your time to die has come.

Death is a natural part of life. From the moment of your birth, you have been dying. You can die peacefully or fearfully, depending on how you live and go through the dying process. If you run away from death, your fears will increase and create more negativity. You are best off preparing for your death and the death of your loved ones.

Before traveling abroad, you decide where to go, how to get there, and what travel documents are required. You figure out how much money is needed and what clothes to pack. If you show up at the airport without reservations and travel documents, you won't be allowed to board your flight. Similarly, now is the time to prepare for death. Getting ready promotes a smooth transition when you and your loved ones die.

Accept Death

The first step in preparing for death is to accept the reality of impermanence. Every family has experienced the death of a loved one. Realizing that death is both real and universal can help you to develop a peaceful mind about leaving your body and current life.

A famous story is told about a young woman who lived at the time of the historical Buddha, about twenty-six hundred years ago. She was married to a rich young man. A son was born to them. Despite their wealth, the boy died when he was a toddler, and she was grief-stricken. She carried her son's dead body from person to person asking for medicine that would restore him to life. People began to think that she was mentally ill.

Someone told her, "Go to see the Buddha. He has the medicine you need." She went to the Buddha and asked for medicine to restore her dead son to life.

The Buddha advised her to obtain some mustard seeds from a family that had not experienced death and bring the seeds back to him. Carrying her dead child, she went from home to home asking for mustard seeds. Everyone was willing to give her mustard seeds, but she couldn't find a single family in which death had not occurred.

She realized that more people had died than were living, and her family was not the only one to experience death. As her attitude changed about her dead son, she no longer felt attached to his body. She returned to the Buddha without her son's body. "I can't find a family that hasn't experienced death," she reported.

The Buddha said to her, "You thought that you were the only person whose child died. Now you realize that death comes to all living beings."

The Buddha explained that life does not end at death. One day of life for a person who accepts deathlessness, he said, is better than one hundred years of life for someone who is afraid of dying. He advised her to meditate on the unsatisfactory, impermanent nature of all phenomena. This advice helped her to develop compassion and wisdom.

As the story illustrates, all living beings die. Everyone is touched by death. Developing peace of mind about this reality cultivates compassion and wisdom.

Create Good Karma

The second step to prepare for death is to create good karma (good energy) during this lifetime. Rather than predestination or fate, karma is a *Sanskrit* word meaning action. An action always produces a result, which in turn leads to another result. Cause and effect are inherent in all phenomena.

Karma is empowering. You create your karma by what you think, say, and do, as well as by what you fail to think, say, and do. Bad karma (negative energy) arises from unethical, negative behavior. You harm yourself, others, and the environment. Good karma results from ethical, positive behavior. You treat yourself kindly and reach out to help others. If you can't help, at least you don't harm.

Good karma produces happiness in life and death. Bad karma causes suffering in life and death. Happiness and suffering aren't accidental but the outcomes of your choices. Because of karma, your thoughts, words, and deeds affect not only you. They produce a ripple effect, like a stone thrown into a pond. Your interest and the interests of others are inextricably connected. By creating good karma, you contribute to the whole.

Heal Your Mind and Life

The third step to prepare for death is to heal your mind and life. That way, you don't have to deal with a troubled mind and bad karma on your deathbed. Root out the three mental poisons. Come to terms with your life. Repair your broken heart and negative memories. Listen to your inner voice and positively reframe your past.

Forgive anyone who you think has wronged you. Moreover, make amends to people you hurt, including yourself. Say "I love you, please forgive me, I forgive you."

Before you experience a health crisis, arrange for someone to take care of you when you no longer can meet your own needs. Designate who will make health-care and financial decisions for you. Explain what health care you want when you are dying, where you wish to die, and what to do with your body after you die.

Complete your legal and financial transactions. Pay your bills. Arrange for your possessions to go to the recipients of your choice and avoid the possibility that your survivors will fight over them. If you put your affairs in order now, you will be able to let go and die when your body and mind are worn out. Otherwise, unfinished business may cause you to hold on to your life and experience a difficult death.

Look deep within yourself. Connect with your best ethical, spiritual values. Fill your life with happiness, love, kindness, compassion, altruism, joy, patience, tolerance, forgiveness, humility, contentment, responsibility, and peace. By training your mind to be positive, you behave virtuously even as your body deteriorates. Your relationships become smooth, and you experience joy. Adversity doesn't affect your tranquility.

Many people die without healing their mind and life, often because they and their families, friends, and health professionals deny that they are dying. What is lost by this denial? The opportunity to become more fully human. In the deepest sense, everyone wants to complete life and die triumphantly.

Negativity during life results in negativity and suffering while dying. On an ongoing basis, heal your conflicts and practice compassion. Then you won't be plagued by unresolved issues. You won't be fearful and remorseful. Instead, you will face death with peace, confidence, and even joy. You will feel grateful that you made a necessary and important contribution to the whole, which is a triumphant way to leave this life.

DEATH

Mindfully Experience Dying

If your mind is clouded, and you fear dying and death, you are likely to suffer on your deathbed. You interpret pain and the dying process from a negative perspective. Rather than be fully awake, you may ask for medications that put you to sleep. You want to be anesthetized from what you are experiencing. The source of suffering is belief in the false dualities of you versus others and life versus death. If you realize the interconnectedness of everything, you will transition smoothly from life to death.

Tibetan medicine, based on Tibetan Buddhism, teaches that an ideal way to die is to be fully conscious. Being alert allows you to experience the dying process. You comfort and thank your loved ones, friends, and health professionals who are taking care of you. While saying goodbye, you give them permission to go on living after your death. You leave them with an invaluable gift by being a role model of how to live and die well.

During your life, train yourself to meditate and breathe properly to calm your mind and body. Then use these practices while dying. Meditation and correct breathing decrease suffering and the need for pain and sleep medicines. If you are alert, you can use the dying process to purify your mind. An accomplished meditator views dying as the ultimate opportunity to gain spiritual realization and a good rebirth or enlightenment.

How to Meditate on Your Breath while Dying

- Lie or sit in a comfortable position with your back straight.
- Lower or close your eyes and relax.
- Engage in circular breathing: Breathe through your nostrils, from your abdomen, slowly, deeply, evenly, with your in-breath the same as the out-breath, and no break in between.
- Focus on your breath: Notice that your breath is warm when you breathe out and cool when you breathe in.
- Count your breaths to stay focused; after you reach ten, go back to one.
- When your mind wanders away, bring it back to your breath.
- If you feel pain, breathe to the pain, rather than trying not to think of it.
- Continue to engage in circular breathing as much as you can to calm your mind and body, oxygenate your tissues, and get rid of toxins.

Recognize Your Impending Death

When you are on your deathbed, people may visit you. You probably won't die right away if you enjoy their visits. Being interested in your visitors and upcoming events, such as a graduation or wedding, may delay your death.

Troubling dreams on your deathbed suggest that you will die soon. These dreams may result from disease obstructing your brain and other parts of your body. Interpreting your dreams in a positive manner can reduce their negative effect.

You will die soon if the nature and treatment of your disorder are the same. The treatment makes the dysfunction worse. For example, you may have a cold imbalance because *loong* and **baekan** are too high and **tripa** is too low. This imbalance intensifies if you are anxious and immobile, and you ingest cold food, beverages, and medications.

Sudden negative changes in your behavior suggest that you will die shortly. For example, you become fearful about others and worry that they will harm you. You develop a dislike for your health professionals, treatments, friends, family, and teachers. Negativity disturbs the three *nyepa* and promotes premature death.

Death is near if you don't respond to treatment, you refuse food, and you develop a putrid body odor. You will die soon if your body stops functioning properly and *loong* no longer flows freely in your channels. Death is likely to come shortly if you lose your physical radiance and become depressed.

Understand Gross Death

Tibetan Buddhism describes two levels of death: gross or coarse death and subtle death. Here are signs of immediate gross death: Your five elements dissolve, lose power, and gradually fade away. Your five senses stop functioning, your heart ceases to beat, and you no longer breathe. You are clinically dead. After your gross death, your subtle death takes place when consciousness separates from your body.

Like all phenomena, you are composed of energy (see chapter 3). *Joongwa-nya* means the five sources of energy from which everything arises. These sources can be understood as five characteristics or elements of energy. Tibetans use a term from nature to describe each element, but element refers to energy, not the usual meaning of **earth, water, fire, air,** and **space**.

During the first stage of gross death, the **earth** element disintegrates, and the **water** element becomes more pronounced. Your vision blurs because of muscle degeneration, and you lose your sight. Externally, your body becomes thin, and your strength diminishes. You feel like you are sinking under the ground. As an internal sign, you may feel as if you are seeing a mirage.

In the second stage of gross death, the **water** element diminishes, and the **fire** element becomes more pronounced. Externally, your body no longer retains moisture, and your body orifices and cavities dry up. You stop feeling physical pain and pleasure, and you no longer hear external and internal sounds. Internally, you may feel like you are engulfed in smoke.

The third stage occurs when the **fire** element decreases, and the **air** element becomes more pronounced. Externally, your body stops being warm, and you are cold. You lose your sense of smell and no longer digest food or beverages. Your inhalation is weak, although your exhalation may be strong and long. You don't remember people's names. As an internal sign, you may see fireflies everywhere.

The fourth stage of gross death takes place when the **air** element lessens, and the **space** element becomes more pronounced. Externally, you stop breathing, your heart ceases to beat, and your brain no longer functions. Your tongue becomes thick and short, and the root turns blue. You no longer are aware of tastes, touch, and your surroundings. Internally, you may experience the appearance of a flickering flame.

Understand Subtle Death

After gross death, you enter the stages of subtle death. Depending on your circumstances and spiritual insight, these stages may last for a moment, a few days, or even several weeks. Your consciousness separates from your body at the end of subtle death. Tibetan Buddhist texts explain these stages for highly evolved practitioners. You can learn more about subtle death by reading these texts and books listed in the bibliography.

During life, experienced spiritual practitioners train in advanced meditation. When dying, they do these practices. They want to be awake and fully experience dying.

Some advanced meditators go through gross death and are declared clinically dead. However, they remain in a meditative state for a few days to several weeks. This highly advanced meditation occurs during the fourth or final, subtle stage of dying and is called "clear-light state," or *chi-way-voe-cel* in Tibetan.

Tibetans use the Tibetan term *thukdam* for this advanced meditation during the last stage of subtle death. An advanced meditator in *thukdam* doesn't breathe, the heart doesn't beat, and the brain no longer functions. Although the practitioner is clinically dead, attendants notice that the person's body doesn't lose moisture and temperature, show signs of decomposition, and go through rigor mortis. Because of preparing well during life, the meditator uses *thukdam* as an opportunity to purify the mind.

How to Help Someone Die Peacefully

If you accept your own death, you are better able to support an individual who is dying. First, though, heal your fears, or you may impose your perspective on the dying person. You inadvertently may keep the individual from dying according to her or his trajectory. By transforming your fears into compassion and wisdom, you can serve as a kind of midwife to help the person die according to her or his own needs and karma.

To provide care, collaborate with the dying person, family, health professionals, and spiritual teachers. Hospice professionals can help you to understand what physical support is needed.

Provide Physical Care for a Person Who Is Dying

- Give prescribed medications to manage pain, and don't be concerned about addiction.
- Teach breathing techniques to reduce anxiety, promote relaxation, and control pain.
- Breathe with the person to help reduce anxiety.
- Offer complementary therapies, such as massage and music the person enjoys.
- Arrange the room to please the individual.
- Provide moisture for dry lips, mouth, and skin.
- Keep the individual's skin clean.
- Change the person's head position to decrease labored breathing.

- Help the individual to maintain proper posture, do passive range of motion, and reposition the person to avoid bedsores and to increase circulation.
- Keep the air fresh, clean, and comfortable; use a humidifier, as needed, to moisten dry air.
- Turn on soft lighting if the person's vision blurs.
- Limit the number of people in the room to avoid confusion and noise.

While doing physical care, provide emotional support. Most important, be a healing presence. Your positive energy will help the dying person to feel safe and loved, to let go of fear, and to cultivate peace. Being a healing presence isn't what you do, but who you are. You are mindfully and kindly in the present moment. Fully attentive, you open yourself to your own and the other person's individuality, strengths, and weaknesses without any judgment.

Provide Emotional Care for a Person Who Is Dying

- Talk in a soothing voice and be reassuring if the person becomes anxious.
- Avoid loud, disruptive expressions of emotion around the individual.
- Create a quiet, peaceful, pleasant atmosphere.
- Provide comfort by touching the person appropriately.
- Avoid minimizing the individual's painful emotions.
- Encourage the person to put legal and financial affairs in order.
- Describe the physical changes that are taking place, as needed.
- Accept that the individual may be angry and view dying as stressful and untimely.
- Allow the person to die in her or his own way, even if the death is challenging.
- Treat the individual with compassion, no matter how she or he behaves.

Besides physical and emotional care, you can offer spiritual care to someone who is dying. You can support the person's efforts to heal the mind, relax into the dying process, and let go. Ethical listening is a powerful way to give spiritual care and offer the opportunity to talk in depth. This kind of listening means to pay full attention to and *really* hear what the person says.

Provide Spiritual Care for a Person Who Is Dying

- Establish rapport by moving closer to and looking softly at the individual.
- Use open-ended communication, such as "Go on," to support the person to uncover hidden conflict, like peeling away layers of an onion.
- Listen quietly, without saying much.
- Encourage the person to talk freely, as needed.
- Avoid lecturing, criticizing, giving advice, or appealing to religious dogma.
- Support the person to let go of negativity, to forgive, and to ask forgiveness.
- Support the person to think about positive memories, love, and happiness.
- Support the person to give permission for loved ones to go on living happily.
- Support the person to develop nonattachment and gratefulness.
- Support the person to treat everyone kindly.
- Support the person to look deep within to ethical, spiritual values and to remember wise guidance from beloved teachers and publications.
- If the dying person is interested, suggest simple meditations that promote relaxation and relieve pain, such as meditation on the breath.

Providing compassionate, appropriate care for a dying person is therapeutic for both of you. Your support gives the individual an opportunity to verbalize feelings and let go of negativity. Talking can uncover deep-seated values, fears, and joys. This ethical, spiritual work promotes resolution of conflicts in a manner that leads to meaning and integrity. Your presence demonstrates that the person is loved and not alone. Awareness and insight transform fear into peace of mind. Being with the person prepares you for your own eventual death.

BARDO: INTERMEDIATE STATE BETWEEN DEATH AND REBIRTH

The Tibetan Book of the Dead (Bar do tö dröl chen mo)

After subtle death, your body no longer functions at any level. Life force has left your body. You are in the bardo, the intermediate stage between death and rebirth. Your subtle consciousness is alive even though it separated from your body.

Bar do tö dröl chen mo is a unique, sacred guidebook and travelogue about each stage through which everyone travels during the bardo. In the eighth century, Padmasambhava (Guru Rinpoche) compiled these teachings in Tibet. His wife, Yeshe Tsogyal, wrote down the teachings. These teachings became *Bar do tö dröl chen mo*, which is translated as *The Great Liberation through Hearing in the Bardo.*[1]

W. Y. Evans-Wenz,[2] with help from Kazi Dawa Samdup, an English teacher at a boarding school in Gangtok, India, translated *Bar do tö dröl chen mo* into English. Evans-Wenz published the book in 1927 under the name *The Tibetan Book of the Dead.* Renowned Swiss psychologist Carl Jung wrote a commentary for the Evans-Wenz translation. Jung explained that *The Tibetan Book of the Dead* was his life's partner because it revealed the secrets of the soul. Since 1927, many translations and editions of the book have been published. These publications are readily available in various languages.

The fundamental teaching of *The Tibetan Book of the Dead* is that all suffering results from belief in a separate self or ego as the center of existence. This self-centeredness isn't caused by innate evil or original sin, but by ignorance about the true nature of existence. If you view yourself as the center of the universe, your egotistical perspective prevents you from understanding reality. The remedy is to see through this illusion. Recognize your false interpretation and dissolve your ego in the light of reality.

Tibetans read *The Tibetan Book of the Dead* as a guide for life, dying, and death. Ideally, during the bardo, they calmly recognize what is occurring and choose a good rebirth or enlightenment. After someone dies, Tibetans chant from *The Tibetan Book of the Dead* to assist the person through the *bardo* to a good rebirth.

Health professionals in some hospices read *The Tibetan Book of the Dead* to individuals on their deathbed. A documentary was made of how a San Francisco hospice uses the book to counsel persons who are dying. To watch this video, go to the YouTube video "*The Tibetan Book of the Dead, Part 1: A Way of Life.*"

How to Go through the Bardo

The Tibetan Book of the Dead describes what occurs during the bardo. Ideally, the dead person lets go of negativity and becomes enlightened. If so, the person is not reborn in *samsara* (cyclic existence of life, death, bardo, and rebirth) but goes on the path to Buddhahood.

For everyone else, the bardo lasts forty-nine days, a number that may be symbolic. During the forty-nine days, Tibetans engage in rituals and chant from *The Tibetan Book of the Dead* to help the dead person travel through the bardo and choose a good rebirth. To watch a docudrama of the bardo, go to the YouTube video "*The Tibetan Book of the Dead, Part 2: The Great Liberation.*"

According to *The Tibetan Book of the Dead*, your consciousness is free from body while you are in the bardo. Without attachment to body, you have the clearest experience of reality of which you are spiritually capable. Everything in your consciousness confronts you, whether these images are negative, positive, or neutral.

If, during life, you purified your bad karma and healed your mind, you experience reality directly. You realize that the images in your consciousness are not real. These projections are empty of inherent existence. Rather than take them seriously, you let them go and choose a good rebirth as a human being. Better yet, you experience your Buddha-Nature. You become enlightened and are liberated from *samsara*.

A different scenario awaits if you did not heal the three mental poisons. Instead, you pushed this negativity deep into your unconscious mind. Now in the bardo, this negativity keeps you from experiencing reality directly. You do not recognize your Buddha-Nature. Terrifying images arise from your troubled mind and propel you to choose an undesirable rebirth.

In both life and death, "demons" in your mind become larger when you run away from them. Unless you realize their emptiness, you believe they are real. If you turn around and face these "demons," they dissolve, just as clouds disappear in the sky.

REBIRTH

Requirements for Rebirth

To be reborn, your subtle consciousness must be attracted, driven by karma and the three mental poisons, to a couple having sex. Ideally, the couple prepared physically, mentally, and spiritually for conception. The mother and father must be in good health and produce a healthy egg and semen. Healthy human menstrual blood is red and odorless; a blood stain easily can be cleaned with washing. Healthy human semen is white in color, heavy in nature, sweet in taste, and abundant in quantity.

Your subtle consciousness enters the mother's ovum as it is fertilized by the father's sperm. The five elements must be present for conception to occur and the embryo to develop. Matter cannot be formed without the **earth** element. Cohesion will not occur without the **water** element. The **fire** element is essential for the embryo to develop heat and functioning internal organs. The **air** element causes the embryo to move and facilitates development. The **space** element is needed for the embryo to have sufficient room to develop into a baby.

The Six Realms of Existence

Your karma determines your state of existence after you are reborn. If you aren't enlightened, you are reborn in one of six realms. Each realm can be an actual physical existence and/or a mind-set. For example, you may be reborn as an animal or as a human being with characteristics of the animal realm. In any realm, you can experience the mind-set of all six realms throughout your life.

The three Upper Realms are preferable to the three Lower Realms. Choosing the Human Realm is essential. You only can become enlightened if you are reborn in the Human Realm and you use your precious human life to cultivate compassion and wisdom.

The Six Realms of Existence

Lower Realms

- **Hell Realm (*Nyal-wa*):** Life devoted to aggression.
- **Hungry Ghosts Realm (*Yi-thak*):** Life devoted to craving.
- **Animal Realm (*Shue-dro*):** Life devoted to gratifying instincts.

Upper Realms

- **Demi-god Realm (*Lha-ma yi*):** Life devoted to quarreling, jealousy, and competition.
- **Human Realm (*Mee*):** Life devoted to a search for meaning and happiness.
- **God Realm (*Lha*):** Life devoted to pleasure and comfort.

The Hell Realm is the lowest state of existence or mind-set. If you are reborn in this realm or develop this state of mind, you use violence to deal with life. Your violent mind-set fills you with hostility and fear. You torture yourself and others, and they torture you.

If you are reborn in the Hungry Ghosts Realm or develop this mind-set, you are obsessed with the past and aren't mindful of the present or future. You feel a terrible emptiness inside that you try to fill in unsatisfactory ways. Constant, insatiable craving and feelings of starvation characterize your life and consciousness.

The Animal Realm lacks the positive qualities of animals. If you are reborn in this state or develop this mind-set, you are obsessed with gratifying instinctual desires for food, drink, and sex. Stupidity and servitude characterize your consciousness and, thus, your life.

When you are reborn in the Demi-god Realm or develop this mind-set, you behave with relentless, competitive aggression. You quickly become angry and jealous. Powerful and fierce, you continuously are at war with yourself and others. Even so, you are better off in this state than in the Lower Realms because you cultivate some positive qualities.

If you choose to be reborn in the Human Realm or develop this mind-set, you experience the precious opportunity to purify negativity and liberate yourself from suffering. Because you consist of both strengths and weaknesses, you have the capacity to feel the full range of emotions from happiness to suffering. You have potential to develop compassion and wisdom, and to bring healing to yourself and the world. By devoting your life to virtue, you can create an enlightened mind, unless you are blinded and consumed by attachments.

Of the six realms, you are most fortunate to be reborn as a human being. To illustrate this teaching, Tibetan teachers tell a story about a turtle swimming in one of the seven oceans on earth while an inner tube floats on one of these oceans. Being reborn as a human being is as unlikely as if the turtle pokes its head through the inner tube's center.

Everyone who is reborn as a human being developed good karma over many lifetimes. Behaving badly, though, burns off good karma. If so, the next time the person is likely to be reborn in a lower realm.

The seductive Realm of the Gods consists of sensual pleasures. If you choose this realm and mind-set, you may become a leader and obtain honor, power, and possessions. Surrounded with grandeur, you live long, but your comfortable life causes you to become egotistical, arrogant, and complacent. The greater your success, the more you suffer from attachments. You cannot be enlightened because you are blind to your own and others' suffering. Next time, you likely will be reborn in a lower realm.

Rebirth and Responsibility

Once you are reborn, you probably won't remember your past lives. Even so, you engage in actions and perceive phenomena by what you were accustomed to in your former lives. The person you are today is an accumulation of all of your experiences during all your lives. Unless you purify your mind, your karma (energy) continues from lifetime to lifetime.

In your new life, you are surrounded by people you knew in previous lives. You will interact with them for many more lifetimes unless you become enlightened. Therefore, your responsibility to others has no beginning or end. Everyone was your mother in a previous lifetime, and you were a mother for everyone else.

When you cultivate this perspective, your heart fills with compassion, and you reach out to help others. You collaborate with others to repair the world, rather than focus on your comfort and success. Eventually, you evolve into a *Bodhisattva*, a highly accomplished spiritual practitioner who is free of suffering and works to liberate all beings from suffering.

Is Rebirth True?

Believing in rebirth may be too big a leap for you. British philosopher John Locke wrote about the difficulty of choosing beliefs. No one knows for sure what happens after death. Investigate beliefs, he advised, and select what makes sense to you and comforts you.

Even if you don't believe in rebirth, these teachings can be helpful for you. Think through what you believe happens after death. Do your beliefs make sense to you? Do they help you to live with meaning and integrity? If not, it's time to cultivate beliefs and values that guide you to create a happy life and a good death.

Wisdom traditions teach three major perspectives on what happens after death. According to one view, "good people" go to heaven and "sinners" go to hell for eternity. This teaching doesn't make sense because no one is simply good or bad. Even if you go to heaven, how will you be happy if your loved ones and other people are in hell?

Other wisdom traditions teach that after you die you cease to exist. Your energy disappears. This teaching isn't consistent with nature.

Tibetan medicine, based on Tibetan Buddhism, teaches a third perspective that is consistent with the natural world. All phenomena are made of energy. When a leaf falls to the ground, its energy doesn't die but transforms into something else. The leaf decomposes into nutrients that help other plants to grow. Similarly, after your body dies, your energy—your subtle consciousness—continues.

You are like an ocean wave. A wave rises for a moment, breaks on shore, and then is gone. This single, identifiable wave has run its course, but water in the wave remains in the ocean. You are part of the energy field. When your body dies, you don't cease to exist. Your subtle consciousness transitions to your next life or enlightenment. This belief will guide you peacefully through life, death, the *bardo*, and rebirth or enlightenment.

TONGLEN MEDITATION WHILE DYING

Tonglen Meditation will help you to create a good life and a good death. In Tibetan, Tonglen means "to give"—*Tong*—and "to take"—*len,* as explained in chapter 3. By doing Tonglen on your deathbed, you will feel useful even if you are dependent on caregivers. You will purify your mind and send compassion to your loved ones, caregivers, and the world.

Tonglen Meditation is therapeutic if you experience pain and suffering on your deathbed. By doing Tonglen, you will transform negativity into compassion and, thus, reduce your suffering. Your dying process will have meaning if you take in the suffering of others and send them compassion.

To do Tonglen on your deathbed, you need to train yourself to do Tonglen during your lifetime. By practicing now, you more easily will do Tonglen when you are dying.

How to Do Tonglen Meditation When You Are Dying

- Lie down or sit in a comfortable position with your back straight, lower or close your eyes, and relax.
- As best you can, engage in circular breathing: Breathe through your nostrils, from your abdomen, slowly, deeply, evenly, with the in-breath the same as the out-breath, and no break in between.
- Notice where you are holding negativity in your body and mind.
- While breathing in, let all your anxiety, anger, confusion, fear, and any other negativity rise to the surface.
- Visualize this negativity as black smoke and breathe it out completely; fill your heart with compassion for yourself.
- Open your heart to the suffering of your loved ones, your health professionals, and all living beings; breathe in this suffering as black smoke into your heart.
- While breathing out, send compassion in the form of white light to your loved ones, health professionals, and all living beings; visualize giving them health, peace, and happiness.
- Keep breathing in suffering and breathing out compassion for everyone.

- At the end of your meditation, gather up all the black smoke you breathed in, and breathe it out completely with no negativity remaining.
- Continue engaging in circular breathing and keep your heart filled with compassion for yourself and all beings.

If you are at someone's deathbed, you can do Tonglen for the person. Tonglen will be comforting and create peace for each of you. As you do Tonglen, synchronize your breathing with the dying person's breathing. Breathe in the individual's suffering and breathe out compassion to the person. Even if you are in a different location from a person who is dying, you can do Tonglen for her or him.

In summary, you were blessed to be born as a human being. Making wise choices will help you to transition peacefully through life, death, the bardo, and rebirth. Ideally, you will use each stage to purify your mind and evolve to enlightenment.

In part A of the book, chapters 1 through 9 explained how to use Tibetan medicine as self-care. Part B of the book addresses how to include Tibetan medicine in your integrative health-care plan. Integrative care provides more healing options than one type of health care alone. To begin this section, chapter 10 describes the context of Tibetan medicine, both past and present, and gives an overview of the *Gyueshi*, the fundamental text of Tibetan medicine.

Part B

TIBETAN MEDICINE IN INTEGRATIVE CARE

• *10* •

Tibetan Medicine Past and Present

$\mathcal{T}$ibetan medicine's origin is as old as Tibetan civilization. The Tibetan Plateau averages three miles high. The earliest inhabitants of Tibet had to deal with many challenges to thrive in the tallest mountains on earth. By watching birds and animals, they learned to use natural resources for sustenance and healing. Their curiosity about nature and desire to overcome suffering prompted them to develop effective, natural treatments. They passed down this knowledge from generation to generation. Many of these timeless remedies are effective today. Tibetan medicine incorporates this accumulated wisdom about using natural resources to heal disease and create health.

One of the world's oldest known healing traditions, Tibetan medicine has been in continuous use since the historical Buddha lived more than twenty-five hundred years ago. Tibetan medicine is based on teachings of Tibetan Buddhism, a branch of Buddhism that flourished in Tibet. Since ancient times, Tibetan medicine has been practiced in Tibet, India, China, Mongolia, Russia, Central Asia, Nepal, and Bhutan. Now Tibetan medicine is moving to the West and incorporating Western science. Given the limits of conventional care, interest in Tibetan medicine is exploding for use in integrative care.

Understanding Tibetan medicine in context is essential to use the teachings and practices as part of integrative care. Otherwise, Tibetan medicine may be reduced to sound bites and simplistic techniques. Misinterpreting and diminishing Tibetan medicine lessens the effectiveness of this profound holistic healing system.

This chapter addresses the context of Tibetan medicine. First, the chapter gives an overview of the long history and twenty-first-

171

century status. Next, the chapter describes the *Gyueshi* (*Four Tantra*), the fundamental text of Tibetan medicine, and gives a synopsis of each *Tantra*. Finally, the chapter lists steps for doing Loving-Kindness Meditation, an essential practice for integrative care that includes Tibetan medicine.

HISTORY OF TIBETAN MEDICINE

Ancient Tibet

Tibetan medicine's historic roots are in *Bon*, an ancient, indigenous healing tradition in Tibet. *Bon* flourished long before Buddhism arrived in Tibet and the present Tibetan script was introduced. According to some sources, Tonpa Shenrag Miwoche, a *Bon* master, was born in Tibet about the time of the historic Buddha. He wrote treatises that became *Bon*'s foundation. His son, Chebu Trishey, helped to develop *Bon*. Besides *Bon*, Tibetan medicine has been influenced by ancient healing traditions in India, China, Persia, Nepal, and Greece.

Fourth-Century Tibet

Tibetan medicine evolved because of dedicated doctors and Tibetan kings who sponsored them. In the fourth century, Lha Thothori Nyentsen reigned as the twenty-eighth king of Tibet. He learned that Indian physicians Biji Gajey and Bila Gajey were visiting Tibet and treating patients successfully. Summoning the doctors to his palace, he asked them to stay in Tibet and share their knowledge. The king gave his daughter, Yidkyi Rolcha, as a bride for Biji Gajey. The princess gave birth to a son, Dungi Thorchokchan, who became famous as the first court doctor in Tibet. For four generations, the sons of Biji Gajey continued the lineage and served as royal physicians for Tibetan kings.

Seventh-Century Tibet

In the seventh century, Songtsen Gampo, the thirty-third Tibetan king, introduced the modern Tibetan script. For the first time, the oral, indigenous Tibetan science of healing was written in the Tibetan script. Chinese princess Wungshing Kongjo of the Tang Dynasty married the Tibetan king and took Chinese medical texts with her to Tibet. The king invited well-known physicians from India, China, and Persia to share with Tibetan doctors their knowledge of healing. These physicians brought with them texts from their medical traditions, which later were translated into Tibetan.

Each physician wrote a treatise that was incorporated into a seven-volume book, *A Fearless Weapon*, for the king. The Indian and Chinese doctors returned home, but the Persian doctor, Galenos, stayed in Tibet and was appointed court physician. He wrote several medical texts that became part of Tibetan medicine.

Eighth-Century Tibet

Yuthok Yonten Gonpo is the most important physician in the history of Tibetan medicine. In the eighth century, he was viewed as the best physician in Tibet and an emanation of the Medicine Buddha. King Trison Deutsen, the thirty-eighth king of Tibet, appointed him to be his court physician. Yuthok traveled to Nepal, Persia, China, and India to learn about other healing traditions. He attracted medical students and established Tanadug, Tibet's first monastic medical college, which no longer exists.

Also, in the eighth century, King Trisong Deutsen invited eminent doctors from India, China, Nepal, Persia, and East Turkistan to Tibet for the "First International Conference on Tibetan Medicine." This conference was held in 728 at Samye Monastery, the oldest monastery in Tibet. Scholars and physicians from various countries attended.

After the conference, Yuthok compiled this accumulated knowledge of medicine in a book, the *Gyueshi*. However, some experts say that the original Sanskrit version of the *Gyueshi* was written during the fourth century, translated into Tibetan, and rewritten by Yuthok. He wrote many books about Tibetan medicine. According to legend, Yuthok lived for 125 years, affirming the wisdom of the teachings. During tumultuous times, Tibetans protected the *Gyueshi* by concealing it inside a pillar at Samye Monastery.

Eleventh-Century Tibet

In the eleventh century, Tibetans rediscovered the *Gyueshi*. Junior Yuthog Yonten Gonpo, thirteenth in the lineage of the elder Yuthog Yonten Gonpo, revised the *Gyueshi* into its present form. The *Gyueshi* synthesizes Tibetans' knowledge of healing with medical knowledge from Greece and healing systems in Asia. Tibetan medicine, as taught in the *Gyueshi*, is a creative integration of healing traditions across centuries and cultures. The *Gyueshi* continues to be the fundamental text of Tibetan medicine.

Twelfth-Century to Sixteenth-Century Tibet

Tibet produced many physicians during these centuries. The doctors developed the teachings and wrote books about Tibetan medicine. In the fifteenth century, Tibetan medicine flourished primarily through two traditions: Jangpa Tradition in northern Tibet and Zurkhar Tradition in southern Tibet. Although both traditions were based on the *Gyueshi*, each one developed its own textbooks, treatments, and methods for identifying medicinal substances and compounding medicines. The two traditions varied due to differences between the north and south in environment, climate, and lifestyle.

Seventeenth-Century Tibet

The Great Fifth Dalai Lama, Jetsun Ngawang Lobsang Gyatso, appointed Desi Sangye Gyatso, a well-known physician, to be regent. During his regency, the Potala Palace was rebuilt and expanded to its current size, the Golden Stupa was built, and Chagpori Medical College was established in Lhasa. The *Gyueshi* was edited and published. The regent wrote many books about Tibetan medicine, including *Blue Beryl* and *Mirror of Beryl: A Historical Introduction to Tibetan Medicine.*

Regent Sangye Gyatso paved the way for seventy-nine medical *thangka* (Tibetan scroll paintings) to be created. From ancient times, Tibetan doctors have used *thangka* to train medical students. Some scroll paintings illustrate anatomy, physiology, and astrology. Others show the development of a fetus, how to make a diagnosis, and what treatments to prescribe. Tibetan doctors accurately identified and diagrammed physiological phenomena even before the microscope was developed in the West.

Twentieth-Century Tibet and India

In 1916, Men-Tsee-Khang, the Tibetan Medical & Astrological Institute, was established in Lhasa under the auspices of the 13th Dalai Lama. He appointed Rev. Khyenrab Norbu to be his own physician, as well as director of both Chagpori and Men-Tsee-Khang. Rev. Khyenrab Norbu wrote many textbooks about Tibetan medicine and trained individuals who became famous doctors of Tibetan medicine. These physicians included Dr. Tenzin Choedrak, Dr. Lobsang Wangyal, and Dr. Yeshi Dhonden, each of whom became a personal physician for the 14th Dalai Lama.

After China invaded Tibet in 1959, the 14th Dalai Lama and thousands of Tibetans fled across the Himalayas to India, Nepal, and other countries. The Indian government welcomed the Dalai Lama and his fellow Tibetans and gave them permission to settle in Dharamsala, India. Dharamsala is a town in the foothills of the Himalayan Mountains near the Indian side of the border with Tibet. The Dalai Lama, in consultation with Jawaharlal Nehru, India's first prime minister, and with support from the Indian government, focused on preserving Tibetan education and culture.

Tibetan schools were established in India to give Tibetan refugee youth access to both traditional Tibetan education and modern education. The Dalai Lama reestablished Tibetan institutions to preserve and promote Tibetan Buddhism and traditional spiritual practices, art, music, and dance. On March 23, 1961, the Dalai Lama re-established the Men-Tsee-Khang, the Tibetan Medical & Astro-Science Institute, in Dharamsala, India, to preserve and promote Tibetan medicine.

During the Chinese Cultural Revolution (1966–1976), Chogpori Medical College was destroyed and not rebuilt. The Men-Tsee-Khang in Lhasa was spared, temporarily closed, and eventually reopened. Chinese authorities arrested and imprisoned famous Tibetan doctors and their students, many of whom died in prison. Some doctors who survived escaped to India with Tibetan medical textbooks and *thangka*. The Chinese Army destroyed ancient, irreplaceable Tibetan medical texts, *thangka*, and medicines.

TIBETAN MEDICINE TODAY

Tibetan Medicine in India

Today the Men-Tsee-Khang in Dharamsala, India, is the largest, oldest organization outside of Tibet to promote, preserve, and practice Tibetan medicine. The Central Tibetan Administration (CTA) in Dharamsala guides and supports this cultural, educational, and charitable institution. The Men-Tsee-Khang consists of many departments.

The Medical College offers students a five-year intensive education, followed by a one- to two-year internship in Men-Tsee-Khang clinics under the supervision of senior doctors. Graduates earn the *Kuchupa* degree, the Men-Tsee-Khang's beginning educational level for practicing Tibetan medicine. After practicing Tibetan medicine for ten years, doctors with the *Kuchupa* degree can take an exam to earn the *Men-Rampa* degree, the advanced level of education. Senior doctors travel around the world to teach Tibetan medicine, do consultations, and engage with health professionals and researchers from other disciplines.

The Pharmaceutical Department uses environmentally sensitive methods to produce and catalog about two hundred kinds of Tibetan medicines and other medicinal products. The Astrology Department educates students to become astrologers and also produces almanacs, calendars, amulets, and astrological charts. Other departments conduct research; document, preserve, and cultivate medicinal herbs; translate and restore texts; publish materials; teach conferences and workshops; and manufacture medicinal teas, lotions, massage oil, and incense, which the Export Office sends around the world.

Men-Tsee-Khang conducts about sixty branch clinics in India and Nepal. The purpose is to improve the health of Tibetan refugees and non-Tibetans, regardless of caste, creed, or color. The doctors give free care or concessions to poor people, monks, nuns, and Tibetans who recently arrived from Tibet. Besides Tibetans, most people who seek treatment at these clinics are Indian or Nepali.

The Men-Tsee-Khang engages in research and other activities with universities in the United States. Emory-Tibet Partnership at Emory University in Atlanta, Georgia, brings together Western and Tibetan Buddhist intellectual traditions. Emory faculty members travel to Dharamsala to teach Medical College faculty and students about

Western anatomy, physiology, science, and research. Medical College faculty teach Tibetan medicine to Emory students in India during an undergraduate study-abroad course about Buddhism.

Since 2001, the Medical College has collaborated with the University of Minnesota's Earl E. Bakken Center for Spirituality & Healing (Bakken Center). Medical College faculty members participate in research, conferences, and other Bakken Center activities. They help to teach two graduate courses, "Traditional Tibetan Medicine: Ethics, Spirituality, & Healing" and "Tibetan Medicine, Ayurveda, & Yoga in India," a study-abroad course in Dharamsala. Bakken Center faculty members teach Medical College faculty and students about Western research and related topics.

Medical College doctors are immigrating to Europe, North America, South America, Australia, East Asia, and other locations. If awarded funding, they study at universities and combine Tibetan medicine with nursing, conventional medicine, anthropology, acupuncture, pharmacy, and other disciplines. In the United States, the biggest Tibetan communities live in New York City and Minnesota. Toronto and Vancouver are home to Canada's largest Tibetan communities.

Tibetan Medicine on the Tibetan Plateau

The Tibetan Plateau has two major Tibetan medical institutions. The Men-Tsee-Khang in Lhasa includes the Medical College, Research Department, Traditional Hospital, and clinics. Tso-Ngon (Qinghai) Arura Tibetan Medical Group (TATMG), at Tso-Ngon (Qinghai) University in Amdo, is the largest Tibetan medicine organization in the world. TATMG has several institutes.

The Tibetan Medical College offers bachelor's, master's, and PhD programs in Tibetan medicine. After earning the bachelor's degree, graduates must pass a national exam and become licensed to practice Tibetan medicine. Faculty developed the first bachelor's degree in Tibetan medicine nursing. Nursing graduates take the same licensing exam as other nurses in Tibet.

The Tibetan Medicine Museum of China and the Tso-Ngon (Qinghai) Tibetan Cultural Museum collect, preserve, display, and research the culture of Tibetan medicine and Tibet. The Tibetan Great Thangka is the largest display at 2,028 feet (618 meters) long and 8 feet (2.5 meters) wide. Four hundred Tibetan artists took twenty-seven years to design and hand paint this giant scroll.

Tso-Ngon (Qinghai) Provincial Tibetan Medical Hospital has one thousand beds and eleven specialty areas. The hospital integrates Tibetan medicine and the latest technology. Graduates of the bachelor's degree in Tibetan medicine nursing provide care for nearly one hundred thousand people annually from the Tibetan Plateau, China, United States, Russia, Japan, Australia, Europe, and other locations. Other institutes use traditional methods and modern technology to make seventy-four kinds of compounded Tibetan medicines; conduct research; analyze new Tibetan medicines; house digitalized information; and collect, restore, and preserve classical medical textbooks.

Standardization, Accreditation, and Licensure

Faculty at the Men-Tsee-Khang in Dharamsala, the Men-Tsee-Khang in Lhasa, and the Tibetan Medical College in Amdo teach students in Tibetan. Students must be fluent in written and spoken Tibetan. Faculty at the Men-Tsee-Khang in Lhasa and Tibetan Medical College in Amdo also speak Chinese to students. The three colleges require applicants to be high school graduates, but a college degree isn't required to enter the basic program in Tibetan medicine.

Standardization, accreditation, and licensure are not yet established outside the Tibetan Plateau. Tibetan medical schools around the world vary in admission standards, quality, length, and graduation requirements. Education to become a Tibetan medicine doctor ranges from an apprenticeship to a PhD in Tibetan medicine.

Levels of Education to Become a Tibetan Medicine Doctor

- Apprenticeship with someone, such as a parent, who practices Tibetan medicine.
- Some attendance at a school that teaches Tibetan medicine.
- Completion of a bachelor's degree in Tibetan medicine from a qualified Tibetan medical college.
- Completion of a bachelor's degree and master's degree in Tibetan medicine from a qualified Tibetan medical college at a university.

- Completion of a bachelor's degree in Tibetan medicine from a qualified Tibetan medical college, ten years of practice, and completion of an exam leading to the distinguished title *Men-ram Pa*.
- Completion of a bachelor's degree, master's degree, and PhD in Tibetan medicine from a qualified Tibetan medical college at a university.

In the United States, a doctor of Tibetan medicine is called a Tibetan medicine practitioner. Some Americans lacking academic credentials claim to be Tibetan medicine practitioners. Qualified individuals who graduated from recognized Tibetan medical colleges are allowed to practice Tibetan medicine in the United States. However, they must follow state laws about unlicensed practitioners of complementary and alternative health care.

For example, 2018 Minnesota Statutes, Chapter 146A,[1] states that unlicensed health-care practitioners in Minnesota cannot call themselves a doctor; puncture the skin; and use treatments, such as acupuncture, covered by Minnesota licensing boards. They must give each client a detailed bill of rights about their qualifications and the client's responsibilities and rights.

GYUESHI: FUNDAMENTAL TEXT OF TIBETAN MEDICINE

At the three Tibetan medical schools described above, the *Gyueshi* is the fundamental text, along with commentaries, clinical experience, research, and theories of health and disease. The English title of the *Gyueshi* is *The Secret Quintessential Instructions on the Eight Branches of the Ambrosia Essence Tantra*. The text is written in verses. Sage Yidlay Kye questions his teacher, Sage Rigpai Yeshi, who replies. This interactive format encourages readers to ponder the questions and answers.

Read the Gyueshi in English

Because the *Gyueshi* was written in Tibetan, only people fluent in written Tibetan could read this classic text. In 2008, the Men-Tsee-Khang Translation Department in Dharamsala, India, first published the

Gyueshi in English. One goal was to standardize and simplify conversion of Tibetan script to Roman script. Now individuals can read this powerful medical, spiritual text in English.

The Men-Tsee-Khang translators spelled Tibetan terms the way they are pronounced (*loong, tripa, baekan*), instead of the Wylie system of Tibetan transliteration (*rLung, mKhris-pa, Bad-kan*). The translators kept key terms in Tibetan to avoid dilution of the meaning. For example, the English translation uses the terms *loong, tripa*, and *baekan*, rather than **wind, bile,** and **phlegm,** as these terms often are translated loosely in English. **Wind, bile,** and **phlegm** do not express the profound meaning of the three primary energies.

Organization of the Gyueshi

The *Gyueshi* consists of the *Four Tantra*: *Root Tantra, Explanatory Tantra, Oral Instruction Tantra*, and *Subsequent Tantra*. These four treatises are organized into eleven sections, four compendia, fifteen categories, and eight branches of Tibetan medicine.

Components of the Gyueshi's Four Tantra

- **Eleven Sections**: Basic Summary, Formation of the Body, Pathology, Behavior Regimens, Dietary Regimens, Pharmacology, Medical Instruments, Maintenance of Health, Diagnostic Approaches, Methods of Healing, and Practicing Physician.
- **Four Compendia**: Pulse and Urine Examination, Pacifying Medications, Evacuative Therapies, and Mild and Drastic External Therapies.
- **Fifteen Categories about Healing**: *Nyepa*, Disorders of the Visceral Organs, Hot Disorders, Disorders of the Upper Body, Disorders of Vital and Vessel Organs, Disorders of the Genitals, Unclassified Disorders, Disorders That Develop Lesions, Pediatric Disorders, Gynecological Disorders, Disorders Caused by Evil Spirits, Wounds, Toxicities, Geriatric Disorders, and Infertility.
- **Eight Branches of Tibetan Medicine:** Whole Body, Pediatric Disorders, Gynecological Disorders, Disorders Caused by Evil

Spirits, Disorders Caused by Wounds, Disorders Caused by Toxic Substances, Geriatric Disorders, and Infertility.

FOUR TANTRA OF THE *GYUESHI*

Root Tantra

The six chapters of the *Root Tantra* give a synopsis of the *Gyueshi*. First, they address how to discuss the teachings. Then they explain theories of health and disease, diagnosis, and treatment. The *Root Tantra* is the essence of the other three treatises. Theories and practices of Tibetan medicine are based on the *Root Tantra*.

To illustrate the teachings, the *Root Tantra* describes three allegorical trees that Tibetan medical schools traditionally have used as teaching aids. The first tree depicts theories of health and disease. The second tree illustrates diagnostic methods. The third tree symbolizes therapeutic approaches.

Tibetan medical students memorize all three allegorical trees. During exams, students build each tree from scratch using wooden blocks and multicolor buttons. At the same time, they recite by memory the corresponding section of the *Root Tantra*.

Each allegorical tree is painted on a *thangka*, a traditional Tibetan scroll painting. Twelve figures are painted across the top. Sage Master Rigpai Yeshi, portrayed as the Medicine Buddha, is in the upper left corner. Next to him is his student, Sage Master Yidlay Kye, depicted as a Buddha. According to the *Gyueshi*, Tibetan medicine emanated from the Medicine Buddha's heart to his follower, also a Buddha. The other ten figures represent various disciples and sages, both Buddhist and non-Buddhist. According to legend, they also were present when the Medicine Buddha taught Tibetan medicine.

Allegorical Tree Representing Health and Disease   This tree, illustrating health and disease, has two trunks. One trunk portrays a healthy person. The other trunk depicts a sick person. The trunk illustrating a healthy individual has three branches, twenty-five leaves, two flowers, and three fruits. These thirty-three components teach that living according to Tibetan medicine promotes health and long life, which in turn produce spirituality, wealth, and happiness. The tree's second trunk depicts a sick person. The nine branches and sixty-three leaves of this trunk portray the causes and conditions of disease.

Allegorical Tree Representing Diagnostic Methods   This tree has three trunks representing the three primary methods of diagnosis: observation, pulse diagnosis, and questioning. The first trunk has two branches that portray observation of the tongue and urine. The three leaves on each branch represent *loong, tripa*, and *baekan* and how they affect the tongue and urine. The second trunk illustrates pulse diagnosis. The three branches represent the differing pulse natures of *loong, tripa*, and *baekan*. The third trunk, questioning, has three branches that show ways of inquiring about disorders involving each of the three *nyepa*.

Allegorical Tree Representing Four Therapies   The four trunks of this allegorical tree illustrate the four categories of treatment: diet, behavior, Tibetan medicines, and accessory therapies. These remedies range from mild to strong. First, Tibetan medicine practitioners prescribe proper diet and then behavior, the essential foundation of healing and health. If diet and behavior don't reverse the imbalance, they prescribe Tibetan medicines and then accessory therapies. In the case of serious illness, practitioners prescribe all four kinds of treatment simultaneously.

Explanatory Tantra

The *Explanatory Tantra* has thirty-one chapters that cover the life cycle of conception, embryology, childbirth, life, and death. The chapters explain the five elements and three primary energies; causes, conditions, and classification of diseases; diagnosis and treatment; properties of medicinal ingredients; and diet and behavior needed for health. The last chapter describes the *Gyueshi*'s Code of Ethics for Tibetan medical students and Tibetan medicine practitioners.

Oral Instruction Tantra

In ninety-two chapters, the *Oral Instruction Tantra* describes how to apply theoretical principles for diagnosing and treating general and specific disorders. The *Tantra* explains in detail the causes, conditions, classifications, signs, symptoms, diagnosis, and treatments for a wide range of health problems.

Subsequent Tantra

The *Subsequent Tantra* has twenty-seven chapters. These chapters explain principles and methods for doing pulse diagnosis and urinalysis, as well as for diagnosing and treating imbalance. Instructions include how to prepare and use various Tibetan medicines and accessory therapies for hot disorders and cold disorders.

LOVING-KINDNESS MEDITATION

As Tibetan medical colleges teach, loving-kindness is essential for health and happiness. Loving-kindness means the heartfelt yearning that all beings experience happiness and the causes of happiness. Cultivating loving-kindness means to let go of self-centered attachment and recognize the lovable qualities in yourself and others.

In Loving-Kindness Meditation, you visualize yourself as being loving toward yourself first and then all beings and the natural world. Doing this meditation regularly heals the three mental poisons and opens the mind and heart.

How to Do Loving-Kindness Meditation

- Sit comfortably in a straight-back chair, on a meditation cushion, or on the floor; or lie on a bed with your arms along your sides.
- Straighten your back so that you can breathe deeply; lower or close your eyes; relax.
- Breathe in a circular manner, through your nostrils, from your abdomen, slowly, deeply, evenly, with your in-breath the same length as your out-breath, with no break in between.
- When you are deeply relaxed and focused, say from your heart:
  - May all beings be well.
  - May all beings be happy.
  - May all beings be peaceful.
  - May all beings be loved.
- If your attention drifts away, gently redirect it back to these affirmations.

After completing this meditation, continue breathing in a circular manner. Bask in your feelings of loving-kindness. Reflect on how you can bring into everyday life the loving-kindness that you cultivated during the meditation.

In summary, this chapter addressed the context of Tibetan medicine. First, the chapter gave an overview of Tibetan medicine's history and current status. Next, the chapter described the *Four Tantra* of the *Gyueshi*, the fundamental text of Tibetan medicine. The chapter ended with Loving-Kindness Meditation, which is crucial for health and happiness.

The next chapter, chapter 11, outlines the *Gyueshi*'s Code of Ethics for practitioners and students of Tibetan medicine. These ethical values are a prerequisite for using Tibetan medicine as self-care and as part of integrative care. Understanding this Code of Ethics will help you to choose an ethical Tibetan medicine practitioner and other health professionals for your integrative-care team. If you are a health professional and live by this code, you can become a true healer.

• 11 •

Tibetan Medicine's Code of Ethics

$\mathcal{T}$ibetan medicine, Tibet's ancient science of healing, integrates ethics, spirituality, and healing. Ethical behavior is essential to evolve spiritually and heal in mind and body. Ethics, spirituality, and healing are interdependent, not separate disciplines. One without the other two is insufficient to create health and happiness.

The *Gyueshi*, the fundamental text of Tibetan medicine, describes a Code of Ethics for Tibetan medical students and doctors, called Tibetan medicine practitioners in the United States. Tibetan medicine can be understood on many levels from superficial to profound. Living by this code is crucial to comprehend the teachings. Behaving ethically creates a peaceful, balanced life. Individuals who cultivate these values *really* see others' suffering. They realize that Tibetan medicine is not just a medical science, but also a daily, personal, life-transforming discipline.

Living by this code will strengthen you to evolve ethically and spirituality. The code will guide you to choose an ethical Tibetan medicine practitioner and other professionals for your integrative health-care team. To maximize the therapeutic potential, select professionals you trust and who mirror your values. This code will help you to be a healing presence.

This chapter gives an overview of the *Gyueshi*'s Code of Ethics for Tibetan medicine students and practitioners. The six core values are intelligence, compassion, commitment, dexterity, diligence, and proficiency in ethics. The chapter explains why people who live by this code can develop a flawless character and become true healers. They even can evolve into sages: individuals who are revered for their compassion and wisdom. Because ethics requires personal balance, the chapter ends with Shaking and Dancing Meditation to harmonize mind and body.

UNSUITABLE AND SUITABLE STUDENTS

Unsuitable Students

According to the *Gyueshi*, some students aren't appropriate to study Tibetan medicine. Unsuitable students can't retain the teachings. Trying to educate these students is a waste of precious resources. Moreover, egotistical, boastful, arrogant students are unsuitable. They look down on others and lack compassion.

Tibetan medicine should not be taught to students who try to acquire the knowledge deceptively through tricky speech. Ungrateful, they behave disrespectfully. They use duplicity to obtain their teachers' work and then take credit for this work.

Tibetan medicine should be protected from students who lack spirituality and insight. Immoderate, they focus on their immediate pleasure without considering the long-term consequences. As the *Gyueshi* states, a crocodile that swallows a precious jewel doesn't pull out the jewel to wear or sell but keeps it stuck inside. Similarly, the teachings must be kept away from students who don't understand their true value.

Unsuitable students do not behave ethically but covet and even try to take other people's wealth and honor. They are poor role models of health and happiness. If these students become Tibetan medicine practitioners, they likely will focus on accumulating possessions and power, not relieving suffering. They raise hopes by making false promises and claiming successes that aren't true. If their predictions turn out to be wrong, individuals under their care are likely to feel angry, discouraged, and hopeless.

Ideally, teachers of Tibetan medicine develop wisdom about how to deal well with unsuitable students, rather than allow them to become practitioners. Teachers with tainted intentions may fail to correct students' unethical, inappropriate behavior. Such teachers are not able to put the teachings into practice for themselves and their students. The *Gyueshi* advocates safeguarding Tibetan medicine from such students and teachers.

Suitable Students

The *Gyueshi* describes students who are appropriate to study Tibetan medicine and become Tibetan medicine practitioners. They are committed to understanding and applying the teachings. They respect their teachers and do not treat them deceitfully.

Suitable students and practitioners of Tibetan medicine generously share their wealth and time, without feeling loss. They distinguish between hypocrisy and altruism. Kindhearted, they consider other people's benefit to be of utmost importance. Protecting Tibetan medicine in this manner causes the teachings to flourish continuously from one excellent student and practitioner to the next one.

CORE VALUES

The *Gyueshi's* Code of Ethics advocates six core values: intelligence, compassion, commitment, dexterity, diligence, and proficiency in ethics. These virtues characterize exceptional Tibetan medicine practitioners who are true healers.

Intelligence

Intelligence is the most important value. Being intelligent means to cultivate open-mindedness, mental stability, and a discerning mind. With these attributes, practitioners can comprehend complicated medical treatises and develop understanding. They combine scientific analysis and intuition to implement appropriate healing practices without fear and anxiety.

Compassion

Practitioners who live by the *Gyueshi's* Code of Ethics behave with compassion, the heartfelt yearning that all beings be free from suffering and the causes of suffering. They cultivate *bodhicitta*, a Sanskrit word for the mind of enlightenment, a mind that is fully conscious and awake.

Bodhi is a Sanskrit word that means awakening or enlightenment. *Citta* derives from the Sanskrit root *cit* and means "that which is conscious." Practitioners who cultivate *bodhicitta* work for the good of all beings.

To develop *bodhicitta*, practitioners go through three phases: preliminary, practice, and engagement. In the preliminary stage, they realize the nature of suffering and cultivate the intention to help distressed individuals. They avoid attachment to what appears to be good and aversion to what seems to be bad.

In the practice phase, they cultivate Buddhism's Four Immeasurables, as described in chapter 6. They behave with loving-kindness, compassion, empathetic joy, and equanimity. Their intention is to become fully awake without obscurations and help others to do the same.

During the engagement stage, they practice Tibetan medicine by the highest standards. They don't hold grudges and don't avoid challenging individuals. Instead, they provide their services without favoring people who praise them or can benefit them.

Commitment

The *Gyueshi* advocates commitment to the ethical practice of Tibetan medicine. Committed practitioners treat their teachers and other health professionals as colleagues and friends rather than competitors. Because they understand Tibetan medicines and treatments, they prescribe them appropriately. They provide the quality of care they give to their own loved ones. The body and body fluids are not distasteful to them. They show respect for medical practices, instruments, treatments, and tests.

Committed practitioners visualize themselves as the Medicine Buddha. For them, the Blue Buddha's medicinal herb and bowl of nectar are precious jewels that heal all disease and meet every need. Before giving Tibetan medicines, they consecrate them by chanting the Medicine Buddha Mantra, as explained in chapter 7. They encourage recipients to picture the medicines being transformed into spiritual energy that heals mind and body. The mind can heal, even if the body deteriorates. Practitioners who are committed to these spiritual practices bring healing to themselves and others.

Dexterity

Ethical practitioners skillfully provide care. Experienced, they quickly and easily perform diagnoses and treatments. Flexible, they adapt to individual needs. They handle medical instruments with expertise and carefully explain the treatments. Compassionate, they communicate in a manner that promotes calmness and insight.

Diligence

Ethical practitioners carefully and persistently provide timely, appropriate care. They don't delay or disrupt needed diagnoses, tests, and treatments. Attentive to their own needs, they are in optimal health. They serve as role models of Tibetan medicine.

To improve care, outstanding practitioners diligently seek excellent mentors. From these guides, they learn different perspectives and applications. Good mentoring encourages them to cultivate patience and a nonmaterialistic attitude. They are grateful for their mentors and do not take advantage of them.

By being diligent, practitioners avoid laziness, an enemy that hinders improvement. They enhance their understanding by engaging in serious discussions with their teachers, mentors, and colleagues. Taking time for contemplation, they integrate into their practice what they learn. They are mindful of what they know and don't know.

Proficiency in Ethics

Practitioners who behave according to the *Gyueshi's* Code of Ethics provide care accurately, enthusiastically, and conscientiously. Before making a diagnosis and prescribing treatment, they take time to understand the problem fully. Cultivating a positive perspective, they communicate honestly, clearly, and kindly.

Rather than select philosophical extremes, ethical practitioners patiently and systematically avoid what is too little, too much, or adverse. They choose a middle way based on Buddhism's Four Noble Truths and Eightfold Path of Ethics (see chapter 7). Through meditation, they transform negativity into compassion and wisdom.

Ethical practitioners go out of their way to help disadvantaged individuals. They create a loving nature toward everyone. If leniency does not work, they kindly set appropriate limits. They resolve conflict in a manner that helps everyone involved to behave with integrity and create a meaningful life. Calm and contented, they inspire others to feel joy amid challenges. They provide care without going against their own core values and good medical practice.

TIBETAN MEDICAL EDUCATION

The *Gyueshi* states that medical students who want to become exceptional Tibetan medicine practitioners must be suitable and cultivate the six core values. Moreover, they need an excellent medical education that combines theoretical knowledge and practical experience. Besides attending classes, the students go on field trips in the mountains where they learn to identify medicinal plants. They find out how and when medicinal plants grow in their natural habitat, how and when to collect them, and how to maintain plants' potency. Faculty members demonstrate how to detoxify poisonous plants and create medicines: They wash and dry the plants, remove harmful coarseness, and compound them into medicines.

Two notable medical colleges offer education that meets these criteria. One school is the Men-Tsee-Khang Medical College in Dharamsala, India. The other school is the Tibetan Medical College at Tso-Ngon (Qinghai) University in Amdo on the Tibetan Plateau.

Sample Curriculum at the Men-Tsee-Khang Medical College, Dharamsala, India

First Year

- **Gyueshi**: *Root Tantra* and *Explanatory Tantra* and its related commentaries.
- **Content memorized**: All six chapters of *Root Tantra*, allegorical trees explained in *Root Tantra*, six chapters of *Explanatory Tantra*, nomenclature of medicinal plants.
- **Supplemental subjects**: Biology, botany, Buddhist philosophy.
- **Practical training**: Identification of medicinal plants and herbs.
- **Nonmedical subjects**: Tibetan prose, grammar, and vocabulary.

Second Year

- **Gyueshi**: *Explanatory Tantra* and *Subsequent Tantra* and its related commentaries.
- **Content Memorized**: Twelve chapters of *Explanatory Tantra*, medicinal plant nomenclature.
- **Supplemental subjects**: Biology, botany, Buddhist dialectics.
- **Practical training**: Identification of medicinal plants and herbs.
- **Nonmedical subjects**: Tibetan grammar and Western scientific research.

Third Year

- **Gyueshi**: *Subsequent Tantra* and its related commentaries.
- **Content memorized**: Fourteen chapters of *Oral Instruction Tantra*, precise location of visceral organs.
- **Supplemental subjects**: Biology, botany, biostatistics, virology, bacteriology, Buddhist texts and philosophy.
- **Practical training**: Mild therapies, identification of medicinal plants and herbs.
- **Nonmedical subjects**: Eloquent Speech of Sakya Pandita's *Nagarjuna's Letter to a Friend on Code of Conduct* and Tibetan astrology.

Fourth Year

- **Gyueshi**: *Oral Instruction Tantra* and *Subsequent Tantra* and its related commentaries.
- **Content memorized**: Seven chapters from *Subsequent Tantra*, bloodletting (venesection) points.
- **Supplemental subjects**: Biology, botany, and Buddhist philosophy.
- **Practical training**: Pulse reading, urine examination, how to deal with patients and prescribe medicines.
- **Nonmedical subjects**: Tibetan poetry, Tibetan astrology, *Nagarjuna's Letter to a Friend on Code of Conduct*, and Western scientific research.

Fifth Year

- **Gyueshi**: Remaining six chapters of *Oral Instruction Tantra*, last chapter of *Gyueshi*, and its related commentaries.
- **Content memorized**: Concluding chapters of *Gyueshi*, allegorical trees in *Gyueshi*.
- **Practical training**: Accessory therapies, anatomy of upper body.
- **Nonmedical subjects**: Tibetan astrology, Tibetan Buddhist philosophy, Western scientific research.

Sixth Year

- Students complete an internship in two branch clinics for at least six months each.
- Senior faculty members supervise them.

Sample Programs Offered by the Tibetan Medicine College Tso-Ngon (Qinghai) University in Amdo on the Tibetan Plateau

Bachelor's Program in Tibetan Medicine: Four Major Areas of Study

- Tibetan Medicine Clinical Practices
- Tibetan Medicine Pharmaceutics
- Tibetan Medicine Management
- Integrative Medicine (Tibetan Medicine and Biomedicine)

Master's Program in Tibetan Medicine: Six Major Areas of Study

- Research on Tibetan Medicine Classical Literature
- Research on Internal Illnesses in Tibetan Medicine
- Diagnosis and Clinical Skills in Tibetan Medicine
- Global Public Health and Tibetan Medicine Prevention
- Tibetan Medicine Pharmaceutics and Clinical Utilization of Tibetan Medicine
- Tibetan Medicine Preparation and Process Methods

PhD Program in Tibetan Medicine: Two Areas of Research Focus

- Tibetan Medicine Classical Literature Research
- Tibetan Medicine Preparation and Process Methods

EXCEPTIONAL, ORDINARY, AND INCOMPETENT PRACTITIONERS

The *Gyueshi* compares and contrasts practitioners who are exceptional, ordinary, and incompetent. Ideally, ordinary and incompetent practitioners recognize their failings. They follow the *Gyueshi's* Code of Ethics and become excellent practitioners.

Exceptional Practitioners

Exceptional Tibetan medicine practitioners are viewed as genuine emanations of the Medicine Buddha. They promptly correct their defects of body, speech, and mind, and they create balance. Sensual pleasures are not important to them because they are devoted to ethical, spiritual practice.

They understand all aspects of the three primary energies: *loong*, *tripa*, and *baekan*. Moreover, they realize why the three mental poisons cause the *nyepa* to go out of balance and give rise to suffering. Because of their insight, they recognize what remedial measures are needed to reestablish balance. They practice with expertise, insight, and compassion, doing their best to heal disease and promote optimal health.

Such practitioners are sensible and courageous when doing consultations, diagnosing illness, and prescribing treatments. Alert and steadfast, they avoid jumping to conclusions. They take time to ask and answer questions in order to understand the situation. Because they *really* listen, they learn about the nature of the imbalance.

Ordinary Practitioners

Ordinary practitioners fall somewhere on the continuum between outstanding and incompetent. They display some qualities of both categories and are inconsistent in their behavior. Sometimes they demonstrate the qualities of exceptional practitioner, but other times they lack ethics and border on incompetence.

Incompetent Practitioners

The opposite of great practitioners, incompetent practitioners are driven by greed and temporary gains. They may even be quacks and use Tibetan medicine as an agent of death. Rather than follow the *Gyueshi's* Code of Ethics, they try to get away with what they can. They lack compassion for themselves and others.

Like individuals traveling on an unfamiliar road, incompetent practitioners don't recognize signs of imbalance and how to reverse it. They reach the wrong conclusions and prescribe therapies that make things worse. If they don't understand the effect of diet and behavior, their treatments may even intensify imbalance and destroy body constituents. Incompetent practitioners ruin people's lives and should be avoided.

REWARDS FOR EXCELLENCE

The *Gyueshi* describes two rewards for behaving according to the Code of Ethics: material rewards and spiritual rewards. Outstanding practitioners are given material benefits because of their ethical behavior and medical practice. More important, they reap the ultimate reward of becoming a *Bodhisattva* and even a Buddha.

Material Rewards

Ethical practitioners thoroughly investigate the health of each individual in their care. Rather than try to fit everyone into one mold, they view each person as unique. Humble and modest, they only accept reasonable payment for services. They are respected for treating everyone, even challenging individuals, with ease and affection.

By cultivating these virtues, ethical practitioners reap the benefits of their devotion to the well-being of others. They are rewarded with affection, gratitude, and praise. Experiencing peace and happiness, they are likely to be blessed with wealth, good health, prosperity, fame, and even reverence.

Ultimate Rewards

Some ethical practitioners abandon all deceitfulness and self-centered-ness. They engage wholeheartedly in service to suffering individuals in a tumultuous world. Motivated by great compassion, they evolve into a *Bodhisattva*, an enlightened being whose intention is to relieve suffering. They generate *bodhicitta*, the spontaneous wish to attain Buddhahood for the benefit of all beings. Ultimately, they can become a Buddha, the unsurpassed state of perfect spiritual awakening and joy.

SHAKING AND DANCING MEDITATION

To become an exceptional person, you, like students and practitioners of Tibetan medicine, are best off living by the *Gyueshi*'s Code of Ethics. Behaving ethically will help you to avoid the turmoil resulting from harmful thoughts, words, and deeds. You can become a healing presence by following the code.

You not only need to behave ethically to evolve into an outstanding individual. Also, you need to keep your mind and body in balance. Shaking and Dancing Meditation will assist you in this ethical, spiritual work.

How to Do Shaking and Dancing Meditation

Preparation

- Turn on a recording of calm, soft music that you enjoy.
- Stand up tall, with your feet flat on the ground.
- Find your own space where you feel comfortable.
- Lower your eyes and go inside yourself.
- Breathe in a circular manner, through your nostrils, from your abdomen, slowly, deeply, evenly, with the in-breath the same length as the out-breath and no break in between.

Shake in Time to the Music

- While breathing in a circular manner, identify negativity in your mind and let it go.

- Identify tension in your body and let it go.
- Shake off all negativity and tension in time to the music.
- Relax your mind and body, becoming one with the music.

Dance in Time to the Music

- While breathing in a circular manner, dance in time to the music.
- Flow with the music.
- Become one with the music, with yourself, and with everything.
- Experience peace, freedom, love, and bliss.

After your meditation, continue breathing in a circular manner. Carry into your everyday life the relaxation and peace you experienced during your meditation. Infuse your life with balance, compassion, and wisdom.

In summary, living by the *Gyueshi*'s Code of Ethics will help you to evolve into an exceptional person. The code will guide you to select outstanding Tibetan medicine practitioners and other professionals to provide your integrative care. If you are a health professional, you will enhance your effectiveness by following the code and becoming a true healer.

However, behaving according to the *Gyueshi*'s Code of Ethics isn't sufficient for integrative care that includes Tibetan medicine. You also need to learn about disease, diagnosis, and treatment according to Tibetan medicine. The next chapter explains how Tibetan medicine practitioners conceptualize disease. Learning about their perspective will expand your thinking and help you to integrate Tibetan medicine into your integrative health-care plan. A combination of Tibetan medicine, conventional care, and other modalities offers more options than only one approach to healing and happiness.

· 12 ·

Disease

Tibetan medicine teaches that health and dis-ease (lack of ease) arise from the same origin. Similarly, water and ice have the same source. Ignorance and its outcome—the three mental poisons—are the distant cause of disease. The immediate cause is the three *nyepa*: **loong**, **tripa**, and **baekan**. Understanding the origin is crucial to prevent, manage, and heal disease and to create health and happiness.

Health is a state of balance. Your *joong-wa-nya*, the Tibetan word for the five elements, or sources of energy, interact harmoniously. As chapter 3 explains, all phenomena are composed of energy that has five sources, translated as elements. To describe them, ancient Tibetans used words from the natural world: **earth, water, fire, air**, and **space**. The five sources or elements are the essence of everyone and everything both outer (environment) and inner (physical body).

Your five elements give rise to your three primary energies, called *nyepa* in Tibetan. The three *nyepa* are further classified into fifteen subtypes based on their physical and mental functions. When you are healthy, your *nyepa*'s current percentages are consistent with their percentages in your constitution. Your **loong**, **tripa**, and **baekan** don't rise too high, fall too low, and/or become disturbed. All fifteen subdivisions of your *nyepa* function properly. You do not disuse, over-use, and or misuse your body, speech, and mind, as explained in chapter 4.

You create health by choosing and properly digesting a diet that supports your constitution. From this nutrition, your body generates seven essential body constituents: (1) nutritional essence that produces (2) blood, that produces (3) muscle tissue, that produces (4) fatty tissue, that produces (5) bone, that produces (6) bone marrow, and that produces (7) regenerative essence. The seven body constituents release

197

three waste products: (1) feces, (2) urine, and (3) sweat (see chapters 5 and 8).

Disease is a state of imbalance in your three *nyepa* and their fifteen subtypes, your seven constituents, and your three waste products. Symptoms of imbalance may take years to appear. You may not recognize them until you come down with a full-blown disease. This chapter explains how Tibetan medicine doctors, called Tibetan medicine practitioners in the United States, view the causes, conditions, location, and characteristics of disease and what you can do to create health. The chapter ends with White Light Meditation to heal mind and body.

CAUSES

Countless variables cause disease. Tibetan medicine organizes them into two categories: distant cause and immediate cause. If practitioners only treat symptoms, any underlying dysfunction may stay hidden and even get worse. To heal the source of imbalance, practitioners identify and treat both the distant cause and immediate cause. The next sections explain the process of developing imbalance and getting sick.

Distant Cause of Disease

Tibetan medicine divides the distant cause of disease into two categories: general and specific. The distant general cause is ignorance about the intrinsic nature of reality. You don't realize that all phenomena consist of energy, and you are part of the energy field, not a separate being. Moreover, you fail to understand that all phenomena are impermanent, empty of inherent existence, dependent on each other, and interconnected.

If you are ignorant of this reality, you spend your life trying to defend your ego that doesn't exist. A bird casts a shadow on the ground no matter how high it soars. Likewise, you can't avoid suffering and disease if you are unaware of impermanence, emptiness, dependent origination, and interconnectedness, as explained in chapter 7.

Tibetan medicine defines suffering as dis-satisfaction (lack of satisfaction). If you hold a materialistic view, you unknowingly try to grasp the self. This egotistical attitude creates self-centeredness. You feel frustrated because no matter how hard you try, you never get enough of what you want, and you can't avoid what you don't want. When you focus on yourself, you end up dissatisfied, and you suffer as a result.

This wrong view about reality produces the distant specific cause of disease: the three mental poisons that, in turn, give birth to the three *nyepa*. Greed, attachment, and desire create and result from *loong*. Anger, hostility, and aggression create and result from ***tripa***. Delusion, confusion, and closed-mindedness create and result from ***baekan***.

Immediate Cause of Disease

The three primary energies, the immediate cause of disease, are essential for life. If, however, they go out of balance, they destroy life. *Nyepa* means fault or defect. Wood illustrates how life-giving *nyepa* retain within them the potential to be defective. Firewood is burned to produce heat for cooking and warmth, but an out-of-control fire destroys everything in its path.

Similarly, ***loong***, ***tripa***, and ***baekan*** carry within them inherent faults. If you engage in the three mental poisons, you disrupt your three primary energies. Your *nyepa* manifest as imbalance that produces suffering and disease.

Under the influence of the three mental poisons, you reach wrong conclusions about how to create health and happiness. Instead, you undermine yourself by engaging in harmful behavior, such as unhealthy choices about your diet, behavior, environment, work, and associates. An unwholesome diet, unethical behavior, inappropriate environment, work you don't like, abusive associates, and other negativity disrupt the three *nyepa*. They rise too high, fall too low, and/or become disturbed, and they go out of sync with your constitution.

Imbalance in your ***loong***, ***tripa***, and ***baekan*** negatively affect your seven body constituents and three excretory functions. Your body cannot nourish itself properly and get rid of toxins. Suffering and disease arise from this state of disequilibrium.

Like everyone else, you were born with a unique constitution that has strengths but also weaknesses. You have vulnerabilities involving your gender, age, stage in life, climate, injuries, lifestyle, microorganisms, and multiple other factors. Your body is aging, and you will die. If the three mental poisons cloud your mind, you are likely to make choices that exacerbate these weakness. To avoid getting sick, you are best off understanding some primary causes of disease.

Some Primary Causes of Disease

- You don't keep your current percentages of *loong*, *tripa*, and *baekan* consistent with their percentages in your constitution.
- You make unhealthy decisions about what to eat and drink, how to behave, where to live, when to sleep, who to emulate, how to support yourself and spend your time, with whom to associate, and so forth.
- You make poor choices that result in injury and fail to treat the impairment properly.
- Your body is wearing out, and you fail to adapt and replenish yourself.
- You deny that you will die and don't prepare well for death.

When one *nyepa* goes out of balance, the other two primary energies are likely to be affected, too. Disease is more serious when your dominant energy is out of balance than if your secondary energies are involved. If, for example, you have a *tripa* constitution and you develop a *tripa* disorder, you likely will get sicker than if you have a *tripa* constitution and come down with a *baekan* dysfunction.

Always, *loong* is part of imbalance. Ordinarily, *loong* goes out of balance first. You feel anxious and can't sleep. *Loong* connects with *tripa* (hot) and *baekan* (cold). *Tripa* causes hot disorders and burns the body constituents. Like the nature of the fire element, *tripa* is hot and flares upward, although *tripa* is in the central part of the torso. Cold disorders develop from *baekan* and reduce body heat. *Baekan* is heavy and cool, like the nature of the earth and water elements. Although located in the upper body, *baekan* tends to flow downward.

CONDITIONS

Tibetan medicine practitioners not only recognize distant and immediate causes of disease. Also, they identify three main conditions that set the stage for illness to develop: (1) progressive condition, (2) arousal condition, and (3) accumulative manifesting condition. You can avoid getting sick by steering clear of and dealing appropriately with these conditions.

Progressive Condition

Inadequate, excessive, and/or adverse seasonal and environmental changes make you prone to illness. For example, inadequate effects result from too little heat in summer, too little cold in winter, and too little rainfall during the rainy season. Excessive effects occur during a sizzling summer, frigid winter, and torrential rainstorms. Adverse effects arise when heat, cold, and rain produce harm.

You become susceptible to disease if you use your sensory organs in inadequate, excessive, and/or adverse ways. Your sensory organs become stressed if you don't use them, such as plugging your ears and putting patches on your eyes. Use of your sensory organs is excessive when you fail to notice what they tell you and adjust your behavior accordingly. For example, you eat food that doesn't look, smell, and taste good, and you get sick. An adverse effect occurs from hurting your sensory organs, such as looking directly at the sun or listening to loud music that damages your hearing.

Leading an inadequate, excessive, and/or adverse lifestyle creates conditions for disease. Your lifestyle is inadequate when you are sedentary and withdrawn. If you try to do too much and deplete yourself, your lifestyle is excessive. Your lifestyle is adverse if you behave unethically, hurting your mind and body.

Arousal Condition

Ideally, you are mindful and avoid the progressive condition. If not, you become prone to developing the arousal condition. You can dodge disease by becoming aware of and staying away from behavior that triggers imbalance in the three primary energies.

Behaviors That Arouse **Loong**, **Tripa**, *and* **Baekan** *Imbalance*

These Behaviors Arouse **Loong**

- You ingest too many foods and beverages with a bitter, light, rough nature, such as drinking too much coffee or eating a fresh arugula salad while drinking iced tea.
- You don't eat regular, nutritious meals.
- You don't routinely sleep deeply and sufficiently at night.
- You overindulge in sex, crying, grief, or anything else.
- You engage in strenuous and/or excessive mental and verbal activities.
- You bleed excessively.
- You have severe diarrhea and vomiting.

These Behaviors Arouse **Tripa**

- You ingest food and beverages with hot, sharp, and oily qualities, such as eating french fries and a spicy cheeseburger while drinking alcohol.
- You nurse anger inside.
- You sleep at noon in hot weather.
- You work too hard and too long, especially in hot weather.
- You exercise strenuously in a hot setting.
- You are injured.
- You are abused emotionally and/or physically.

These Behaviors Arouse **Baekan**

- You ingest foods and beverages with bitter, sweet, heavy, cold, oily qualities, such as drinking iced tea with a cold sandwich, potato salad, and carrot cake.
- You nap during the day or immediately after a heavy meal.
- You sleep in a damp, cool environment.
- You become chilled after swimming.
- You wear clothes that aren't warm enough.
- You eat and drink too much.
- You eat a meal before digesting your previous meal.

Accumulative Manifesting Condition

If an imbalance is aroused and you don't reverse it promptly, you are likely to experience the accumulative manifesting condition. This dysfunction worsens, displays symptoms, and even spreads to other body locations. You are sick. Arousal, accumulation, and manifestation may occur instantaneously or take place over decades. For example, a viral or bacterial infection may seem to appear suddenly, but cardiovascular disease may take many years to develop.

Loong accumulates from a diet of rough, cold foods and beverages. For example, you frequently eat raw salads while drinking iced coffee or iced tea. To pacify *loong*, ingest what is oily and warm, such as buttered wheat toast and warm soup.

Tripa accumulates from ingesting sharp, hot foods and beverages. Examples are eating deep-fried, oily foods while drinking alcohol. To pacify *tripa*, ingest what is astringent and cool, such as cool banana pudding and cool herbal tea.

Baekan accumulates from a heavy, oily diet of cold foods and beverages. For example, you eat a cheeseburger and fresh green salad with salad dressing, and you wash them down with iced tea. The cold drink reduces digestive heat and causes fat in the cheeseburger and salad dressing to solidify, producing indigestion. Qualities of roughness, warmness, and lightness pacify *baekan*. Examples are steamed, warm fish and slightly cooked vegetables seasoned with salt and lemon.

When the progressive and arousal conditions exist, weather can create an accumulative manifesting condition. *Loong* tends to accumulate during rainy, cloudy, windy, cool weather. Sunny, humid, warm weather pacifies *loong*. *Tripa* accumulates in humid, rainy, hot weather. Cool, dry weather pacifies *tripa*. Overcast, cold, damp weather causes *baekan* to accumulate. Sunny, warm, dry weather pacifies *baekan*. To avoid getting sick, live and work in an environment that supports your constitution.

LOCATION

Besides identifying the causes and conditions of disease, practitioners of Tibetan medicine identify the site(s) of the disorder in the body. This analysis requires understanding the interdependent nature of the five elements, three *nyepa*, seven constituents, and three waste products. Knowing the location of the dysfunction sheds light on which *nyepa* are out of balance and how to reverse this dysfunction.

The primary location for **loong** is in the torso below the navel, particularly in the colon. Moreover, **loong** is prevalent in joints, bones, skin, and ears. **Loong** disorders arise in these sites.

Tripa primarily is in the torso between the navel and the heart. **Tripa** imbalance occurs in this location. Also, **tripa** dysfunction arises in the blood, sweat glands, eyes, and skin.

Baekan primarily is located above the heart. **Baekan** imbalance occurs in the chest, throat, lungs, head, site of undigested food, muscle tissue, fat, bone marrow, regenerative fluid, feces, urine, nose, and tongue. Discomfort in these areas may indicate a **baekan** dysfunction.

CHARACTERISTICS

Along with determining the cause, conditions, and location, Tibetan medicine practitioners diagnose characteristics of the disease. This task becomes challenging if more than one *nyepa* is out of balance. Characteristics of a dysfunction indicate which *nyepa* has risen too high, fallen too low, and/or become disturbed.

For example, **loong**, **tripa**, and **baekan** work together to produce digestive heat essential for digestion. Eating a hot, spicy diet increases digestive heat, which is harmful for a **tripa** constitution. Regularly ingesting a cold diet decreases digestive heat and increases indigestion, which aggravates **loong** and **baekan** constitutions.

To avoid getting sick, you are best off learning the characteristics of excessive, deficient, and/or disturbed **loong**, **tripa**, or **baekan**. Developing awareness will help you to reverse any imbalance right away. Two or all three of your primary energies may be affected. If so, you will exhibit the symptoms of whatever *nyepa* are not in sync with your constitution.

*Characteristics of Excessive, Deficient, and/or Disturbed **Loong***

*Excessive **Loong***

- Thin physique with a darkening complexion.

- Longing for warmth.
- Tremors, dizziness, loss of strength.
- Abdominal distention and constipation.
- Nonstop talking.
- Insomnia.
- Improper functioning of the internal organs.

Deficient Loong

- Lack of energy and loss of interest in talking.
- Physical discomfort.
- Unclear memory.
- Symptoms similar to an excess of **baekan**.

Disturbed Loong

- Empty, floating pulse.
- Transparent water-like urine that becomes lighter after transformation.
- Inability to sit still.
- Unstable, fluctuating, irritable mental disposition.
- Dizziness, tinnitus.
- Dry, reddish, rough tongue with astringent taste in the mouth.
- Shifting, strong pain that spreads with movement; sharp pain in the back of the neck, chest, and/or jaws.
- Rigidity and contraction, as if the body is restricted, but wanting to stretch the limbs.
- A feeling like the waist, hips, and other joints are battered, muscle and skin are parted, and bones are breaking.
- Cold feeling accompanied by shivering and goosebumps.
- Lack of energy.
- A feeling like the eyes are bulging.
- Insomnia, but frequent yawning and sighing.
- Tender **loong** points, such as at the temples.
- Dry heaves, vomiting of soft bubbly sputum, abdominal distention and rumbling.
- Symptoms most apparent at dawn, dusk, and after food is digested.

Characteristics of Excessive, Deficient, and/or Disturbed **Tripa**

Excessive **Tripa**

- Yellowing of feces, urine, skin, eyes.
- Increased hunger and thirst.
- Elevated body temperature.
- Itching.
- Darkening of skin or white patches.
- Diarrhea.
- Frequent anger and hostility.

Deficient **Tripa**

- Decline in body heat and brightness of complexion.
- A feeling of cold.
- Indigestion.
- Lethargy.

Disturbed **Tripa**

- Overflowing, thin, twisted, fast pulse.
- Urine that is reddish-yellow in color and has a foul smell with a lot of steam.
- Headaches.
- Body heat.
- Sour-bitter taste in the mouth.
- Thick coating on the tongue.
- Reddish-yellow sputum with a salty taste.
- Dry nostrils.
- Reddish-yellow sclera.
- Localized pain.
- Less sleep at night and uncontrollable sleep during the day.
- Extreme thirst.
- Presence of blood and bile in diarrhea and vomitus.
- Profuse sweating with an unpleasant odor.
- Reddish-yellow complexion.
- Symptoms most apparent at noon, midnight, and during digestion of food.

*Characteristics of Excessive, Deficient, and Disturbed **Baekan***

Excessive **Baekan**

- Decrease in body heat.
- Indigestion.
- Lethargy and sense of heaviness in the body.
- Pale complexion.
- Excessive saliva and sputum.
- Heavy sleep.
- Breathing problems.

Deficient **Baekan**

- Dizziness.
- Trembling of the heart.
- Laxness of the joints.
- Flabby, loose limbs.

Disturbed **Baekan**

- Sunken, weak, slow pulse.
- Whitish urine, with less odor and steam.
- Loss of the sense of taste.
- Paleness of the tongue and gums; whitening of the sclera.
- Excessive nasal discharge and sputum.
- Confused mind and unclear memory.
- Feeling of heaviness of mind and body.
- Loss of appetite and poor digestion.
- Loss of body heat.
- Pain around the kidneys and waist.
- Swelling of the face and body; weight gain.
- Development of a goiter.
- Presence of undigested food and mucus in the feces and vomitus.
- Sleepiness, lethargy, procrastination.
- Tightness and stiffness of joints.

- Symptoms most apparent during the rainy season, at dusk, in early morning, and immediately after eating.

Any imbalance affects the whole body. Excessive, deficient, and/or disturbed *nyepa* harm the seven body constituents. The body loses the ability to get rid of toxins in the three waste products. The body constituents and waste products go into a state of excess or deficiency. By being aware of these characteristics, you can reverse them before they get worse.

Characteristics of Excess and Deficiency in the Body Constituents

Nutritional Essence

- Excess is like the symptoms of excess in **baekan**.
- Deficiency causes emaciation, difficulty swallowing food, rough skin, discomfort.

Blood

- Excess leads to cancer of the visceral organs; disorders of spleen, blood, and **tripa**; jaundice; gingivitis; difficulty with physical movement; reddening of eyes, urine, skin.
- Deficiency produces laxity of blood vessels; rough skin; yearning for cool, sour food.

Muscle Tissue

- Excess causes goiter, inflammation of lymph glands, increase in body weight.
- Deficiency leads to joint and limb pain, and adherence of skin to bone.

Fat

- Excess causes tiredness, enlargement of the breasts, abdominal fat.

- Deficiency results in less sleep, emaciation, a pale bluish complexion.

Bone and Bone Marrow

- Excess causes too much bone development, too many teeth, sense of heaviness in body, impaired vision, joint enlargement.
- Deficiency leads to loss of hair, nails, teeth.

Regenerative Fluid

- Excess produces pathological formation of mineral concretions, such as kidney stones, and increase in sexual desire.
- Deficiency results in bleeding and burning sensations in the genitals.

To function well, the seven body constituents must get rid of toxins through their waste products. Excessive and deficient feces, urine, and perspiration poison the body. Vitality suffers and produces emaciation, loss of physical radiance, fearfulness, and depression. *Loong* that rises too high has similar characteristics. Nutritious foods, such as milk and warm soup, are remedies to restore vitality and decrease *loong*.

Characteristics of Excess and Deficiency in the Waste Products

Feces

- Excess leads to heaviness in the body, abdominal distension, intestinal rumbling.
- Deficiency causes intestinal flatulence with rumbling sounds and upward movement of *loong* that produces pain in the ribs and heart.

Urine

- Excess causes pain in the urethral orifice and unsatisfactory urination.

- Deficiency leads to urine discoloration, difficulty in urination, scanty urine.

Perspiration

- Excess causes profuse sweating, unpleasant body odor, skin diseases.
- Deficiency results in cracking of skin and loss of body hair.

CREATE HEALTH

Experienced practitioners of Tibetan medicine are able to diagnose imbalance before diagnostic tests in conventional care indicate abnormality. You will create health by consulting periodically with these practitioners. Moreover, regularly complete the Constitutional Self-Assessment Tool (CSAT) and Lifestyle Guidelines Tool (LGT) explained in chapter 2. Use this information to reverse any imbalance promptly and avoid getting sick.

The five elements and three *nyepa* are the very source of your existence. Your unique combination of **loong**, **tripa**, and **baekan** forms the framework of who you are. By freeing yourself from ignorance, you transform the three mental poisons into wholesome choices that support your constitution. You create health and decrease the causes of disease.

The ideal time to reverse imbalance is when it first begins. Promptly notice any discomfort and take steps to make things right. Mindfulness will help you to heal imbalance, rather than wait until disease develops. The more you learn about how your body functions, the better choices you will make to avoid and/or heal disease and to create health.

Choose your diet carefully and digest your food well. When you ingest food and beverages, pervasive **loong** spreads the qualities in your body. Too much or too little of these qualities can cause imbalance. Unless you reverse the imbalance, the disorder accumulates and progresses like the buildup of clouds before rain. Eventually, the disorder manifests, courses through its pathways, and becomes disease.

Throughout your life, countless variables bombard you. If you develop clear thinking, you will make healthy choices that decrease your vulnerabilities, or at least keep them from sabotaging you. You will transform your weaknesses into strengths.

Even if you make healthy decisions, though, your body is mortal and eventually will break down. You don't need to suffer if you are injured, you get sick, and/or your body wears out. Suffering begins in the mind. Disease is an opportunity to retreat from everyday life and figure out why you got sick. Purify your mind and cultivate compassion and wisdom. No matter what your health status is, you can create a healthy, peaceful mind.

WHITE LIGHT MEDITATION

The five sources of energy, fifteen subdivisions of the three *nyepa*, seven body constituents, and three waste functions each have the potential to develop imbalance. Even so, all disorders have the same nature: They result from ignorance, the three mental poisons, and imbalance in **loong**, **tripa**, and/or **baekan**.

White Light Meditation will help you to transform the three mental poisons into positive thinking that creates health and happiness. Doing this meditation will energize you and heal your mind, even if your body is deteriorating, and you are on your deathbed.

How to Do White Light Meditation

- Sit comfortably in a straight-back chair, on a meditation cushion, or on the floor; or lie down with your arms along the sides of your body.
- Straighten your back so that you can breathe deeply, but don't cross your legs, or your energies may not flow freely.
- Lower or close your eyes and relax your entire body.
- Breathe in a circular manner, through your nostrils, from your abdomen, slowly, deeply, evenly, with your in-breath the same length as your out-breath, and no break in between; keep breathing in this manner throughout the meditation.
- Visualize a pure, white light above the crown of your head.

- Feel the light wash over the top of your head, forehead, back of your head, cheeks, eyes, face, neck, shoulders, arms, hands, and fingers.
- Feel the light become stronger and more vibrant as it washes over your heart center, abdomen, back, hips, legs, feet, and the bottom of your feet.
- Feel the light all around you and inside you; become one with the light.
- Let all of your negativity come to the surface and breathe it out.
- Feel purified and energized in mind and body.

When you are ready, open your eyes. Continue breathing in a circular manner. Bring into everyday life the purity and energy you cultivated during the meditation.

This chapter explained how practitioners of Tibetan medicine understand the causes, conditions, location, and characteristics of disease, as well as how you can create health. These teachings are too complicated for one chapter. Even so, this overview will help you to become mindful about the nature of disease and how to include Tibetan medicine in your integrative health-care plan.

Practitioners of Tibetan medicine not only must understand health and disease, but they must make accurate diagnoses. The next chapter explains diagnosis from the perspective of Tibetan medicine. You will learn how to consult with a Tibetan medicine practitioner as part of your integrative health care.

• *13* •

Diagnosis

$\mathcal{I}$n Tibetan medicine, an experienced doctor of Tibetan medicine, called a Tibetan medicine practitioner in the United States, is the gold standard for constitutional analysis. The practitioner graduated from a qualified Tibetan medical college and developed diagnostic expertise under the mentorship of senior practitioners. The person behaves according to the *Gyueshi*'s Code of Ethics and treats everyone with skill, compassion, and wisdom.

As part of your self-care and integrative care, you need to learn about your constitution and current state of your *nyepa*. You can do this analysis by completing the Constitutional Self-Assessment Tool (CSAT). Then you can use the Lifestyle Guidelines Tool (LGT) to create a plan for living in harmony with your constitution, as explained in chapter 2. However, studies suggest that most people don't know themselves well enough to do accurate self-assessments. You likely will increase the accuracy of your assessment by combining the CSAT, LGT, and a consultation with an excellent, experienced practitioner of Tibetan medicine.

Choose an expert, kind practitioner who tries to understand you. If you feel lonely and undervalued, you are prone to getting sick. Select someone who engages in personal self-healing. To be a healer, the practitioner must heal herself or himself. Pick someone you trust to maximize the therapeutic relationship.

This chapter explains how to prepare for your Tibetan medicine consultation and what to expect. During a consultation, the practitioner uses a systematic diagnostic process and three examination techniques: observation, touch, and questioning. After collecting physiological and psychological information, the practitioner condenses and classifies this content to diagnose health and disease. The chapter ends with a meditation to transform anger, one of the three mental poisons, into compassion, which is essential for health and happiness.

HOW TO PREPARE FOR YOUR CONSULTATION

You can increase the accuracy of the Tibetan medicine practitioner's diagnosis by preparing for your consultation. During the twenty-four hours before your consultation, don't use prescription or over-the-counter medicines unless you will develop health issues without them. For example, keep taking insulin if you have insulin-dependent diabetes. Reduce stress. Engage in circular breathing. Calm your mind and life. Relax to lower your blood pressure and heart rate. Sleep well. Ingest an appropriate, nutritious diet. Be happy.

With these behaviors, you are more likely to create a peaceful mind and balanced *nyepa*. If your mind is disturbed, your three primary energies likely are out of balance. The practitioner may have difficulty identifying your constitution. The two of you may reach wrong conclusions about your constitution and the state of your health.

Activities to Avoid for Twenty-four Hours before Your Tibetan Medicine Consultation

- Foods and beverages that are difficult to digest.
- Foods, beverages, and vitamins that discolor the urine, such as beets and Vitamin C.
- Caffeine, alcohol, drugs, tobacco.
- Excessive sweets, fatty foods, highly spiced foods.
- Sexual activity.
- Thinking and talking excessively.
- Insomnia.
- Sedentary lifestyle.
- Vigorous physical exercise, such as jogging or doing hot yoga.
- Anything else that may affect your *nyepa* and pulse.

Complete the CSAT several times. Learning about Tibetan medicine and doing the CSAT with someone who knows you well can help you to assess yourself accurately. If your CSAT results vary, select the result that you think fits you best. Then use this CSAT result to do the LGT. During your consultation, discuss your CSAT and LGT results and how they compare with the practitioner's analysis of your constitution.

Write down questions to ask the practitioner. Here are sample questions:

1. What is my inborn constitution?
2. What, if any, energies are out of balance?
3. How can I bring my energies back into balance?
4. How can I live in harmony with my constitution?

Include questions about your health issues. List medications you take and why you take them. Leave enough room to take notes on what the practitioner tells you. After your consultation, you can refresh your memory by reading your notes. As with any professional, expect help but not miracles.

On the morning of your consultation, obtain your clean catch, midstream urine specimen. Collect your urine right after you get out of bed in the morning before you eat or drink anything. Your first urine in the morning isn't as affected by digestion as is your urine after you eat and drink. At your consultation, give the specimen to the practitioner.

Obtain Your Clean Catch, Midstream Urine Specimen

- Wash your hands with soap and water.
- Use an antiseptic wipe or soap and water to clean from front to back (females) or from top to bottom (males) the area around the opening of your urethra.
- Begin urinating and then collect your urine midstream.
- Use a clear, clean container, such as a plastic water bottle, that won't change or hide the color of your urine; the practitioner needs to identify the color of your urine.
- Cover your urine and place the container in a paper bag to protect your privacy.

- Don't refrigerate your urine, but keep it out of the sun and in a cool environment.
- Give your container of urine to the practitioner at your consultation.

Before going to your consultation, take a shower to clean your skin and remove perspiration odor. Avoid taking a hot shower or cold shower that can affect your temperature, pulse, and blood pressure. Brush your teeth and clean your mouth and tongue.

Likewise, the practitioner can increase accuracy of diagnosis by preparing for twenty-four hours before your consultation. Preferably, the practitioner avoids stress, drugs, alcohol, spicy food, oily food, and vigorous exercise. Moreover, the night before your consultation the practitioner ideally sleeps well and creates a calm, focused, kind mind.

SYSTEMATIC DIAGNOSTIC PROCESS

During your consultation, the practitioner uses a systematic diagnostic process to investigate your mental and physical health. This process consists of four phases: (1) foundation of investigation, (2) objects of investigation, (3) criteria of investigation, and (4) methods of investigation.

First, the practitioner investigates your *nyepa*, the foundation of investigation. During this phase, the practitioner identifies your constitution and what, if any, energies are out of balance. Chapter 1 lists the seven general constitutions of Tibetan medicine.

Second, the practitioner focuses on the objects of investigation: the state of your five sensory organs, their ability to fulfill their functions, and the five wastes. The five sensory organs are eyes, ears, nose, tongue, and skin. Their functions are to see, hear, smell, taste, and feel. The five wastes are sputum, feces, vomitus, urine, and blood.

The third diagnostic phase consists of seven investigation criteria. If your *nyepa* are out of balance, the practitioner assesses your (1) environment, (2) the season and weather, (3) your age and stage in life, (4) the nature of the imbalance, (5) when your symptoms first appeared, (6) the aftereffects of foods and beverages you ingest, and (7) the location of the disorder in your body. The practitioner uses this information to evaluate the effects of your diet, behavior, and any medicines or therapies you use.

According to karma, each cause yields a corresponding effect. The nature of an imbalance corresponds to its cause. As stated in chapter 12, the practitioner diagnoses a dysfunction by determining its arousal condition and variables that caused it to arise. The relationship between a disorder and symptoms is like the relationship between fire and smoke. Just as smoke implies the presence of fire, symptoms suggest imbalance. The practitioner avoids an inaccurate diagnosis, such as mistaking smoke for steam.

During the fourth phase of the diagnostic process, the practitioner mindfully uses three examination methods: observation, touch, and questioning. These techniques help the practitioner to collect psychological and physiological information about your mind and body. An experienced practitioner skillfully uses these methods.

OBSERVATION

The first method of examination is observation. You walk into the consultation room fully clothed and don't undress. The practitioner observes your appearance: your gender, age, gait, energy, posture, weight, height, and so forth. Going deeper, the practitioner looks at the nature, size, texture, and color of any abnormalities. She or he visually checks the color and texture of your skin, eyes, and nails. If you are sick, the practitioner observes the color and texture of any blood in your feces, sputum, and/or emesis.

The practitioner asks you to stick out your tongue. A healthy tongue is red, smooth, moist, and flexible. If you have a *loong* constitution and/or a *loong* disorder, your tongue is reddish, dry, small, and coarse in texture. Your tongue is long with a thick, yellowish coating if you have a *tripa* constitution and/or a *tripa* imbalance. When you have a *baekan* constitution and/or a *baekan* disease, your tongue has a whitish, sticky, lusterless, moist coating, and a smooth texture. With a dual constitution and/or a dual disease, your tongue shows characteristics of both affected primary energies.

Next, the practitioner checks your urine. Urine is like a mirror that reflects health and imbalance. The practitioner holds up the urine container to see the true color of your urine. Sunlight is best because artificial light can give a false color. Shaking the container, the practitioner looks at the steam, scum, sediments, and bubbles. After removing the cover, she or he smells your urine.

If you are healthy, your urine has a clear, light-yellow color and a slight smell. The vapor is of moderate intensity and duration. The sediments are light and properly dispersed. The higher your body temperature, the more sediments appear in your urine.

Scum that forms on the surface of healthy urine resembles scum on a stagnant pond. The bubbles are moderate in size and uniformly dispersed. As steam evaporates, the bubbles disappear from the periphery toward the center. After this transformation, the urine is clear and whitish yellow. Unhealthy urine is the opposite of these qualities.

If you have a *loong* constitution and/or disorder, your urine is whitish/blue like spring water and has unstable steam. Large bubbles appear as the practitioner shakes or stirs your urine. *Loong* urine smells like undigested food. The sediments are like hair. The scum is scattered.

A *tripa* constitution and/or imbalance produces yellowish-red urine with a foul odor and thick, long-lasting steam. When the practitioner shakes or stirs the urine, tiny bubbles appear and then disappear quickly. The sediments are like cotton thrown in water. The scum on top is thick.

Your urine is white in color if you have a *baekan* constitution and/or imbalance. *Baekan* urine has little odor and light, quick-disappearing steam. When the practitioner shakes or stirs the urine, the bubbles are similar to bubbles in saliva. The sediments are like tips of hair. The scum on the surface is thin.

TOUCH

The second method of examination is touch. The practitioner asks to touch you to identify the temperature, softness, and hardness of your body. If you have an abnormality, the practitioner may ask to touch it to assess its nature. Touch helps the practitioner to assess the quality and location of sensitivity and pain in your body.

In Tibetan medicine, pulse reading is the most important diagnostic method involving touch. Tibetan medicine practitioners devote a great deal of time to developing expertise in and insight about pulse diagnosis. Your body carries energy messages about what is going on inside you, in your environment, and in the cosmos. Your thoughts, diet, behavior, the sun, moon, and multiple other variables affect your pulse, which is like a messenger traveling around your body collecting information about your health. The practitioner accesses this information by palpating your radial artery at each wrist. Your pulse is a messenger between you and the practitioner.

The best, most accurate time for pulse diagnosis is early in the morning before you get out of bed, exhale your warm breath, and inhale cool air. In early morning, your *nyepa* are more likely than later in the day to be in a balanced state. Your pulse and respirations aren't yet affected by your activities of taking a shower, getting dressed, and eating breakfast.

However, a practitioner isn't likely to do a consultation before you get out of bed. Therefore, you need to go to the practitioner's consultation room. Ideally, you arrive early and sit quietly before your consultation. Otherwise, your breathing, heart rate, and blood pressure may be high because of traveling to see the practitioner. Do circular breathing to bring your breathing, heart rate, and blood pressure to normal.

If you are female, the practitioner examines your right wrist pulse first. He or she examines your left wrist pulse first if you are male. The practitioner's right hand checks your left wrist, and the left hand checks your right wrist. The index finger, middle finger, and ring finger read your radial artery on one wrist and then the other one. The index finger is just below the first crease in your wrist. The fingers are in a line by one another, yet not touching each other. The practitioner applies small pressure with the index finger, more pressure with the middle finger, and most pressure with the ring finger.

A practitioner experienced in pulse diagnosis can identify your constitution, as well as the state of your internal organs and surrounding tissues. The practitioner's index finger probes the pulses of your lungs, heart, small intestine, and large intestine. The middle finger feels the pulses of your spleen, stomach, liver, and gall bladder. The ring finger examines the pulses of your reproductive organs, kidneys, and urinary bladder.

A *loong* constitution produces a floating, empty pulse with intermittent, halting beats. A *tripa* constitution gives rise to a fast, overflowing, twisting pulse with taut beats. A ***baekan*** constitution causes a sunken, slow pulse with weak, declining beats. A dual constitution shows pulse characteristics of both dominant primary energies.

Your constitutional pulse may be female, male, or neutral. This designation doesn't correspond to gender but to characteristics of the pulse. A female may have a female, or male, or neutral pulse. Moreover, a male may have a male, or female, or neutral pulse. A female pulse is thin and fast, and a male pulse is thick and bulky. A neutral pulse is smooth and flexible.

An experienced practitioner can identify other pulses. Your seasonal pulse, related to astrology, reflects solar-lunar influences on you and the environment. The number of times your life-force pulse beats consistently equals the number of years in your life span. The pregnancy pulse ordinarily is protruding and rolling and may indicate whether the fetus is a female or male. The death pulse has changing characteristics and pauses in pulse. Your various pulses help the practitioner and you to understand who you *really* are.

Through pulse diagnosis, an experienced practitioner can diagnose imbalance before you have overt symptoms and abnormalities appear in conventional diagnostic tests. You are healthy if your pulse beats five times during each of the practitioner's one hundred respirations. If your pulse beats faster, you have a hot disorder. Beating less than five times indicates a cold imbalance.

A hot disorder causes a strong, overflowing, rolling, fast, taut, firm pulse. A cold dysfunction gives rise to a weak, sunken, declining, slow, loose, empty pulse. Generally, a hot imbalance is associated with ***tripa***, and a cold disorder is related to ***baekan***. Neutral ***loong*** can be hot or cold, depending on if it is influenced most by ***tripa*** or ***baekan***.

The pulse of a combined ***loong*** and ***tripa*** disorder is empty and fast. The pulse of a combined ***loong*** and ***baekan*** disease is empty and slow. The pulse of a combined ***tripa*** and ***baekan*** dysfunction is twisted and sunken.

In Tibetan medicine, pulse diagnosis is a complex art and science related to astrology. Excellent practitioners meditate, study astrology, and work closely with astrologers. They develop insight about how the cosmos affects the body, mind, relationships, and environment.

QUESTIONING

Asking in-depth questions is the third examination method of the systematic diagnostic process. The purpose is to (a) determine if and why your *nyepa* are out of balance, (b) identify the disorder's location, and (c) learn about your symptoms. To *really* understand, the practitioner sits near you and listens carefully to you without distraction. The practitioner won't think you are healthy if you are anxious, angry, and/or confused.

The practitioner asks about your health history and causes, symptoms, and sites of any illness. Next, the practitioner makes inquiries about treatments and medicines you use, who prescribed them and why, and how effective they are. Going deeper, the practitioner asks about your diet, behavior, lifestyle, environment, and state of mind. These questions and your responses uncover relevant information about the state of your health.

To diagnose a *loong* disorder, the practitioner asks if you often yawn, stretch your limbs, and/or feel chilled. Do you have pain in your joints and waist and, if so, does the pain stay in one site or shift around your body? Other symptoms of a *loong* imbalance include anxiety, insomnia, irregular lifestyle, and nausea. You may feel uncomfortable after ingesting raw vegetables and other light, rough foods, and you feel better after eating warm, oily, nutritious foods.

To uncover a *tripa* imbalance, the practitioner asks if you regularly ingest a diet that is sharp, oily, and hot in nature, such as fried and spicy foods, while drinking alcohol. Do you feel better after you ingest a cool diet and participate in cooling activities? The practitioner asks about your behavior and whether you push yourself beyond your limits. Are you prone to anger? Do you frequently get headaches, upper back pain, fevers, inflammations, infections, skin rashes, belching, acid reflux, and a bitter taste in your mouth?

When suspecting a *baekan* imbalance, the practitioner asks if you often feel cold. Are your senses dull? Do you feel heaviness in mind and body? How often do you procrastinate and fail to get things done? When stressed out, do you tend to withdraw, rather than interact with others? After eating, are you uncomfortable and feel like your stomach is bloated? A *baekan* disorder is confirmed if you feel better after ingesting warm foods and beverages and engaging in other behavior that heats you up.

CLASSIFICATION

During your consultation, the practitioner uses a systematic diagnostic process that includes observation, touch, and questioning. The purpose is to collect information about the state of your mental and physical health. The practitioner condenses and classifies this information according to the categories below.

Balance or Imbalance

The practitioner classifies your information according to balance or imbalance in your *nyepa*. If you are healthy, the current percentages of your ***loong***, ***tripa***, and ***baekan*** are about the same as their percentages in your constitution. Your three primary energies, seven body constituents, and three waste products function well. You have potential to live a long happy life.

If you have an imbalance, the current percentages of your ***loong***, ***tripa***, and ***baekan*** are not in sync with your constitution. Your three *nyepa* have risen too high, fallen too low, and/or become disturbed. They are not functioning well with your five elements, seven body constituents, and three excretions. Each *nyepa* is associated with specific organs and parts of your body. Any imbalance in a *nyepa* affects the corresponding organs and tissues of your body.

Loong, *Tripa*, *and/or* *Baekan*

If you have a disorder, the practitioner classifies your symptoms according to which primary energy is out of balance. Identifying imbalance is challenging if more than one *nyepa* is not in sync with your constitution. ***Loong***, ***tripa***, and ***baekan*** affect each other. If one energy goes out of balance, the other two energies are likely to go out of balance, too, and create complex diseases that are challenging to reverse.

Causes, Conditions, and Location

The practitioner classifies the imbalance according to what caused it, the conditions that set the stage for it, and its location in your body. Multiple causes and conditions lead to imbalance, as described in chapter 12. The disorder can be in one site or spread to several sites of the body and develop into full-blown disease.

Hot or Cold

The practitioner determines if the disorder is hot or cold. Cold disorders require hot treatments, and hot imbalances need cold therapies. **Loong** and **baekan** are cold in nature and related to the moon. **Tripa** is hot like the sun, as are its corresponding disorders. Although **baekan** clearly is cold, **loong** is harder to understand because it can be neutral. **Loong** is involved in all dynamic processes of health and disease. Therefore, **loong** can intensify **tripa** and **baekan** disorders, as well as pacify imbalance in **tripa** *or* **baekan**.

Simple or Combined

The practitioner distinguishes between simple and combined disorders. The imbalance is simple if only one *nyepa* is out of balance. A simple disorder is independent and only manifests symptoms of imbalance in one primary energy.

In a combined disorder, two or all three *nyepa* are involved. An imbalance with a dependent nature, such as a **loong** dysfunction, combines with one or more other disorders. One imbalance may develop on top of, underneath, or by an existing disorder. For example, cancer is a combined disease with all three *nyepa* affected. That's why reversing cancer is complicated. A cancer may consist of both hot and cold disorders. Cooling the hot imbalance can aggravate the cold imbalance and vice versa.

Prognosis

The practitioner classifies a disease by its likely outcome. The *Gyueshi* explains four categories of prognosis: (1) minor, transient illnesses that heal on their own (*tar-nang-trel-nay*); (2) diseases caused by disturbed *nyepa* that can be fatal but healed with appropriate remedies (*yong-dup-tsey-nay*); (3) imbalances caused by external factors, such as evil spirits, that require healing with spiritual practices (*kung-tak-dhon-nay*); and

(4) fatal disorders, resulting from negative actions in past lives, for which treatment shows little or no effect (*shen-wang-nyon-lay*).

Using categories to classify information helps the practitioner to understand your mental and physical health. If you are sick, the practitioner assesses balance versus imbalance of your **loong**, **tripa**, and **baekan**; which *nyepa* are affected; the cause, conditions, and location of the disorder; whether the disorder is hot or cold and simple or combined; and the prognosis. Appropriate classification is crucial for a correct diagnosis.

Tibetan medicine practitioners recommend at least three consultations. Your **loong**, **tripa**, *and* **baekan** normally rise and fall because of your thoughts, stage in life, what you eat and drink, time of day, weather, stress, and multiple other factors. These variables can cause your *nyepa* to rise too high, fall too low, and/or become disturbed. Having at least three consultations helps the practitioner and you to recognize and understand these changes. Working together, the two of you can identify any imbalance and how to reverse the negative trajectory.

MEDITATION ON ANGER

Tibetan medicine teaches that thoughts impact health and happiness. Kind thoughts calm mind and body. They help you to think clearly and make good decisions.

In contrast, anger increases the heart rate and blood pressure and depresses the immune system. When you are angry, you breathe in a shallow, erratic manner. You get too hot, which affects your entire body. Your cells fail to let go of toxins and become properly oxygenated. Angry thoughts decrease your ability to see things clearly and choose wisely. Anger can kill you.

Meditating on anger will help you to develop mindfulness, awareness of the present moment. When mindful of your anger, you more easily will let it go, rather than express it, ruminate on it, and/or suppress it. Hidden anger comes out in depression, headaches, infections, inflammations, skin rashes, and other symptoms. By meditating on anger, you figure out why you are angry. You can root it out and behave with compassion and wisdom.

How to Meditate on Anger

- Sit comfortably in a straight-back chair, on a meditation cushion, or on the floor; or lie on a bed with your arms by your sides and your legs stretched out.
- Straighten your back and breathe deeply; close or lower your eyes and relax.
- Breathe in a circular manner, through your nostrils, from your abdomen, slowly, deeply, evenly, with your in-breath the same length as your out-breath, and no break in between; keep breathing in this manner throughout the meditation.
- Think of a situation about which you are angry and fully feel your anger; determine where in your body you are holding anger and why.
- Try to understand your anger and what underlies this negativity.
- Do you feel abused? If so, how can you kindly set limits and protect yourself?
- Are you afraid of losing something you have or not getting what you want? If so, remember the folly of being attached to what is impermanent (see chapter 7).
- Did someone disrespect you and you defended your ego to save face? If so, keep in mind that you are empty of inherent existence, and your ego doesn't *really* exist (see chapter 7).
- Breathe out your anger, fear, and all other negativity; feel purified in mind and body.
- Fill yourself with compassion toward yourself, everyone and everything.

When you are ready, fully open your eyes and keep breathing in a circular manner. Bring into your everyday life the purity, peace, and compassion that you cultivated during the meditation. Make amends for treating yourself and others with anger. Kindly set appropriate limits to protect yourself from individuals who are angry. Anger is contagious. If you don't safeguard yourself, you are likely to become angry again.

In summary, this chapter explained how exceptional Tibetan medicine practitioners do constitutional analysis and diagnose health status. They use a systematic diagnostic process and three examination techniques: observation, touch, and questioning. Classifying the resulting physiological and psychological information helps them to understand the nature of any imbalance. An accurate diagnosis is essential to determine what, if any, treatments are needed.

Tibetan medicine practitioners not only must be excellent diagnosticians, but they also must prescribe appropriate remedies to reverse or at least manage imbalance. The next chapter explains treatment from the perspective of Tibetan medicine. Learning about treatment, in addition to disease and diagnosis, will help you to consult with a practitioner and use Tibetan medicine as part of your integrative health-care plan.

• *14* •

Treatment

$\mathcal{A}$fter diagnosing imbalance, Tibetan medicine practitioners prescribe treatment. They consider both mind and body, or the three mental poisons may sabotage healing. Therapy in Tibetan medicine addresses the whole person, not just symptoms of dysfunction.

Countless remedies exist. All phenomena consist of the five sources of energy: **earth**, **water**, **fire**, **air**, and **space**, as explained in chapter 3. Therefore, everything is potential poison or potential medicine. The body, disorders, and therapy are all interrelated because they are based on the five sources of energy, often called the five elements.

Practitioners classify treatment into four categories: diet, behavior, medicines, and accessory therapies. First, they prescribe proper diet and behavior, the essential foundation of health and happiness. If diet and behavior don't reverse the imbalance, they prescribe medicines and then accessory therapies. For a serious illness, they simultaneously prescribe all four treatments: diet, behavior, medicines, and accessory therapies. As the *Gyueshi* states, this intensive approach is like confronting an enemy face-to-face in a narrow alley.

When designing a treatment plan, practitioners follow three steps: (1) Identify the treatment goal, (2) select a suitable remedy, and (3) determine prognosis. Without this systematic process, the *Gyueshi* states, prescribing therapy is like shooting an arrow in the dark and not seeing the target. This chapter explains the treatment goal, the four categories of therapy, and prognosis. Finally, the chapter describes Meditation on Sound, a practice that helps to reverse imbalance and promote healing.

TREATMENT GOAL

Loong, *Tripa,* *and/or* *Baekan*

Balance produces health and imbalance leads to dis-ease (lack of ease). During a consultation, a Tibetan medicine practitioner determines if the person's *nyepa* have risen too high, fallen too low, and/or become disturbed. *Loong, tripa,* and *baekan* go out of balance for many reasons. The goal of treatment is to reverse the underlying imbalance, eliminate symptoms, and heal both mind and body.

Practitioners prescribe cool remedies for hot maladies and warm therapies for cold ones. *Loong* alone or connected to *baekan* is cold, but *loong* connected to *tripa* aggravates hot disorders. Because *tripa* is hot, *tripa* imbalance is hot. Hot illnesses indicate that *tripa* is affected. *Baekan*, which is cold, produces cold diseases. Cold dysfunction results from imbalance in *baekan* alone or together with *loong*.

Using warm and cool therapies improperly exacerbates illness and may even be fatal. For example, warming activities, such as engaging in vigorous exercise or eating too much seafood, intensifies *tripa* (hot) disorders, such as infections, inflammations, and skin eruptions. A *loong* and/or *baekan* dysfunction worsens from cooling behavior. Examples are overeating, a sedentary lifestyle, and eating raw/cold foods. The person may gain weight and develop diabetes.

Loong imbalance is the crucial factor in disorders of the heart, life channel, and colon. *Tripa* imbalance contributes most to liver, blood, and gallbladder dysfunction. *Baekan* is prevalent in stomach, spleen, and kidney diseases.

Simple or Combined Disorder

Practitioners diagnose an imbalance as simple or combined. In a simple disorder, only one *nyepa* is affected. A simple dysfunction usually stays in its site of the body. The treatment goal is to reverse the imbalance before it becomes a combined disorder.

Usually, *loong* goes out of balance first. If it isn't reversed, *tripa* and/or *baekan* are likely to become affected, too. Ideally, practitioners treat a *loong* dysfunction when it first manifests to prevent *tripa* and/

or **baekan** from going out of balance. Oily, warm qualities reverse **loong** dysfunction, whether or not **tripa** and/or **baekan** are involved.

In a combined disorder, two or all three primary energies are out of balance. Over time, improper diet and behavior intensify a simple imbalance. The dysfunction spreads to another body location that already is disturbed, producing a combined disorder. The treatment goal is to reverse the most severe problem to prevent a life-threatening disease. Ideally, treating the critical imbalance heals the secondary one.

Combined disorders, such as cancer and cardiovascular disease, require bringing all three **nyepa** into balance. This task is challenging because **loong**, **tripa**, and **baekan** affect each other. To harmonize all three **nyepa**, treatment must possess both hot and cold qualities.

Wrong therapies can cause combined disorders. For example, practitioners may reduce or strengthen only one **nyepa** in a combined disorder. All three primary energies may become affected and develop even more dysfunction. Incorrect treatment makes any imbalance worse.

DIET

Diet is the first line of treatment. Practitioners prescribe nutritious foods and beverages that support the person's constitution and affected **nyepa**. An unwholesome diet is the primary cause of imbalance. Most health problems around the world can be traced directly or indirectly to an improper diet. Examples of diet-related disorders are alcoholism, digestive issues, hypertension, cardiovascular disease, obesity, and diabetes.

The Six Tastes

Understanding the underlying basis of the six tastes is a key means through which practitioners design a dietary regimen. A daily, nutritious diet includes all six tastes: sweet, sour, salty, bitter, pungent, and astringent. A substance with two or more tastes is categorized according to the basic taste. Each taste is composed of two sources of energy, or elements: **earth, water, fire,** and **air.**

Energy Sources Comprising Each of the Six Tastes

Six Tastes	**Five Energy Sources (Elements)**
1. Sweet	**Earth** and **Water**
2. Sour	**Earth** and **Fire**
3. Salty	**Water** and **Fire**
4. Bitter	**Water** and **Air**
5. Pungent	**Fire** and **Air**
6. Astringent	**Earth** and **Air**

Each of the six tastes has a specific nature and potency resulting from its composition of elements. The six tastes pacify or aggravate the three *nyepa*. Tibetan medicine practitioners prescribe tastes to reverse the imbalance. They avoid tastes that aggravate the imbalance.

Sugar, molasses, honey, butter, and *ghee* (clarified butter) taste sweet. A sweet diet builds the body's constituents and strength, which is crucial for children, elders, and people with a weak body. The sweet taste relieves throat infections and coughs, acts as an antiseptic, and brings a healthy glow to the skin. Sweets increase clarity of the sense organs, promote longevity and rejuvenation, and are an antidote to toxins. Ingesting too many sweets decreases digestive heat, enlarges the glands, leads to obesity, and causes goiters and urinary tract disorders.

Yeast, curd, lemon, and buttermilk are sour. Foods and drinks with a sour taste improve appetite and digestive heat. They aid digestion, decrease phlegm, and satisfy the mind. Too much sour taste gives rise to blood and **tripa** disorders, a flaccid body, contagious illnesses, blurred vision, dizziness, and thirst.

The salty taste reduces body stiffness and clears bowel obstructions and blocked energy channels. Salty, warm compresses generate body heat and induce sweating to remove toxins. Salt improves heat, thirst, and appetite. Excessive salt reduces physical strength and contributes to baldness, grey hair, wrinkles, blood disorders, and edema.

Kale, arugula, bitter gourd, eggplant, and turmeric taste bitter and are an antidote to toxins related to weak liver function. The bitter taste improves appetite, quenches thirst, treats fainting and vomiting, and heals contagious diseases. In addition, the bitter taste enhances mental alertness and treats breast disorders and voice obstruction. The bitter taste in excess weakens body constituents and dries up mucus, fats, oils, bone marrow, feces, and urine.

The pungent taste in dried ginger, black pepper, and some chili peppers treats throat problems, diphtheria, joint pain, and wounds. Pungent ingredients increase body heat, digestive heat, and appetite. They cleanse and open the body channels. Ingesting too many substances with a pungent taste reduces sperm, weakens physical strength, and causes tremors, body contractions, fainting, and pain in the waist and back.

The astringent taste in avocados, raw bananas, cranberries, pomegranates, and pears pacifies blood disorders, replenishes skin color, and heals wounds. In excess, the astringent taste decreases the amount of feces, causes mucus accumulation, and blocks energy channels. Too much astringent taste can lead to abdominal distenion, heart disorders, and the wasting away of body constituents.

After ingestion, a taste is converted into a post-digestive taste upon contact with digestive heat and digestive functions of *loong, tripa,* and *baekan.* The post-digestive taste of sweet and salty ingredients is sweet. The sour taste remains the same after digestion. Bitter, pungent, and astringent tastes change into bitter post-digestive taste. Table 14.1 summarizes how the six tastes affect *loong, tripa,* and *baekan.*

Table 14.1.   How the Six Tastes Affect the Three Primary Energies

Taste	*Loong*	*Tripa*	*Baekan*
Sweet	Pacifies	Pacifies	Aggravates
Sour	Pacifies	Aggravates	Pacifies
Salty	Pacifies	Aggravates	Pacifies
Bitter	Aggravates	Pacifies	Aggravates
Pungent	Aggravates	Aggravates	Pacifies
Astringent	Aggravates	Pacifies	Aggravates

Hot or Cold

Practitioners determine if an imbalance is hot or cold in nature and then prescribe the opposite dietary therapy. Cool foods and beverages reverse a hot disorder. Warm foods and drinks treat a cold dysfunction. For specific foods and beverages, see chapter 8 and the Lifestyle Guidelines Tool in chapter 2.

Generally, plants are hot in nature if they grow in direct sunlight and a southern exposure. These plants pacify cold disorders. Examples are lemons and black pepper. Conversely, plants tend to be cold in nature if they grow in a northern exposure, in shade, or underground. These plants treat hot disorders. Examples are root vegetables, such as potatoes.

Potatoes and other plants with the quality of **earth** (cold) aggravate *baekan* and pacify *loong*. Cucumbers and other plants with the quality of **water** (cold) aggravate *baekan* and pacify *tripa*. Plants, such as chili peppers, with the quality of **fire** (heat) aggravate *tripa* and pacify *baekan*. Lettuce and other leafy plants with the quality of **air** (movement) aggravate *loong* and pacify *baekan*.

Diet to Treat a **Loong** Disorder

Loong imbalance usually develops first. Then this dysfunction disturbs the other two *nyepa*. A diet that promptly reverses a *loong* dysfunction and promotes digestion can prevent the other two *nyepa* from going out of balance, too.

To treat a *loong* imbalance, Tibetan medicine practitioners prescribe a diet that raises digestive heat, particularly during *loong* times of the twenty-four-hour period: 3–7 a.m. and 3–7 p.m. (see chapter 4). The stomach is like a field responsible for the growth of all body constituents. Increasing digestive heat can heal *loong* issues. A warm, nutritious diet strengthens digestive heat and pacifies *loong*.

Strengthening the body treats disorders in which *loong* is too high and the other *nyepa* and body constituents are depleted. Early summer is an ideal time to build up the body. *Loong* disorders are most often seen in elders, pregnant and postpartum women, and persons with insomnia, depression, coughing up of blood, and/or excessive bleeding. Overindulging in sex and/or physical activity can produce *loong* imbalance.

To heal such *loong* disorders, practitioners prescribe a diet with sweet, sour, and salty tastes and that has oily, smooth, and warm qualities. Examples are warm soup, cooked vegetables with *ghee* (purified, clarified butter) or olive oil, most meats (except for pork and goat), molasses, garlic, onion, and milk. Ingesting sesame oil and/or rubbing sesame oil on the skin pacifies *loong*, even if *loong* is combined with a *tripa* and/or *baekan* disorder.

Diet to Treat a **Tripa** *Disorder*

To heal a *tripa* imbalance, practitioners prescribe a cooling diet. Examples are fresh greens, bitter gourd, potatoes and other root vegetables, curd and buttermilk from cows or goats, barley or wheat porridge, and cool water. Normally *tripa* rises from about 11 a.m. to 3 p.m. and 11 p.m. to 3 a.m. Cooling remedies are crucial during *tripa* times.

Diet to Treat a **Baekan** *Dis-order*

Practitioners treat a *baekan* disorder by recommending warm foods and beverages. Examples are spicy chilis, cooked vegetables, mutton, fish, honey, and boiled water with ginger. *Baekan* is highest from about 7 a.m. to 11 a.m. and 7 p.m. to 11 p.m. A warming diet is most important then.

Elevated *baekan* can lead to obesity, diabetes, cancer, lymph node disorders, mental dullness, and increased sputum. Remedies are to lose weight by ingesting only small portions of light, nutritious, easy-to-digest foods and beverages. Don't sleep after a heavy meal to avoid developing a fatty body. Because being lean is preferable to being overweight, eat and drink with discipline and moderation.

Ingesting less foods and beverages treats indigestion, high fat intake, stiff joints, contagious diseases, cancer of the visceral organs, gout, and arthritis. Small portions benefit people with spleen, larynx, brain, and/or heart dysfunction. Restricting food intake is a remedy for tropical diarrhea, vomiting, lethargy, loss of appetite, constipation, urine obstruction, and combined disorders of *baekan* and *tripa*. Winter is the best time for slimming treatment. Fasting is only recommended for individuals who are physically and emotionally strong.

Diet to Treat a Combined Disorder

Practitioners prescribe a diet to reverse a combined imbalance. For example, warm, nutritious foods and beverages build up the body and bring both *loong* and *baekan* into balance. Fasting can heal the simultaneous excess of *baekan* and *tripa* and a deficiency of *loong*. Ingest cool, nutritious foods for combined disorders of *loong* and *tripa*. Cool, light qualities are remedies for combined disorders of *baekan* and *tripa*. Cool, nutritious, light qualities treat combined disorders of all three *nyepa*.

BEHAVIOR

Reverse Imbalance

If dietary changes alone don't heal symptoms and imbalance, practitioners prescribe behavior as treatment. Most important, breathe properly. Anxiety produces shallow, erratic breathing that doesn't remove toxins and oxygenate cells. In contrast, circular breathing calms and replenishes mind and body. Train yourself to breathe in a circular manner. All of the meditations in this book use circular breathing.

Practitioners recommend specific behaviors to reverse imbalance. For example, calm mind and body, such as sitting quietly, to heal *loong* dysfunction. Do what is cooling, such as avoiding the hot sun, to reverse *tripa* dysfunction. Treat *baekan* imbalance with warming activities, such as vigorous exercise. For other specific behaviors, read chapter 8 and the Lifestyle Guidelines Tool in chapter 2.

To reverse imbalance, practitioners prescribe behavioral treatment for the mental poisons. Greed, attachment, and desire cause and are caused by *loong*. The therapy is to meditate on and accept impermanence. Anger, hostility, and aggression cause and are caused by *tripa* and remedied by meditating on and cultivating compassion. Confusion, delusion, and closed-mindedness cause and are caused by *baekan*. The treatment is to meditate on and develop wisdom. A positive attitude strengthens the immune system.

Develop Mindfulness

Practitioners advocate mindfulness to recognize and meet the body's natural needs promptly. Avoid suppressing hunger, thirst, vomiting, sleep, sneezing, yawning, breathing, sputum, tears, feces, flatulence, urine, and sperm. Imbalance and disease result from not meeting these needs.

Suppressing hunger causes emaciation, weakness, anorexia, and dizziness. To recover, eat small quantities of light, oily food, such as warm soup with buttered wheat toast. Engage in warm, peaceful behaviors and create calm, enjoyable relationships.

Suppression of thirst causes a dry mouth, dizziness, heart disease, and mental illness. A remedy is to ingest a cooling diet, such as vegetables and non-caffeinated beverages. Engage in cooling activities, such as walking safely in nature.

Suppression of vomiting causes loss of appetite, breathing problems, generalized edema, cancer, eye dysfunction, and increased sputum. To heal, don't eat until the urge to vomit goes away. Gargle gently and use calming aromatherapy and herbal tea.

Sleep suppression can cause yawning, lethargy, heaviness of the head, and indigestion. Holding back yawns and sneezing leads to headaches, stiff neck, facial palsy, jaw dysfunction, and unclear sensory perceptions. To treat them, use aromatherapy, nasal drops, and warming up in the sun.

Suppressing breathing after exertion harms both mind and body. Tumors, heart disease, and mental disturbance can develop. After exertion, rest and breathe deeply as needed. Let your breathing, blood pressure, and heart rate return to normal.

Retaining sputum increases sputum. Complications are asthma, weight loss, hiccups, heart disease, and anorexia. Cough or spit out phlegm from the throat and lungs.

Withholding tears can lead to heart disease, headaches, dizziness, anorexia, and a runny nose. Let the tears flow and figure out why you are crying. Then heal your broken heart. Change what you don't like— or come to accept it. Meditation, sleep, and talking with people you trust can transform sadness into gratefulness.

Suppressing flatulence and feces can cause intestinal blockage, constipation, hard bowel movements, abdominal cramps, and halitosis. Retaining urine can produce kidney stones and disorders of the urethra, penis, and pelvis. The body may become toxic. Tumors, blurred vision, low body heat, heart disease, headaches, calf muscle cramps, and the common cold may occur. To heal, take medicinal baths, have oil massages, use compresses, and ingest medicinal butter.

Retention of sperm can lead to involuntary ejaculation, urinary obstruction, penile ache, calculi formation, and impotency. Remedies are sex, mild enemas, and medicinal baths. Ingesting milk, chicken, or herbal tea can bring relief.

When natural urges are suppressed, *loong* becomes disturbed, and many kinds of disorders arise. Symptoms may lessen with time. However, a relapse is likely unless *loong* is pacified. Besides the above therapies, use treatments for *loong* imbalance.

Create a Peaceful, Happy Life

A peaceful, happy life reverses imbalance. Practitioners prescribe relaxation techniques to nurture mind and body. Listen to beautiful music, flowing water, and other pleasant sounds. Do gentle yoga postures. Exercise appropriately. Unwind before bedtime and sleep soundly.

Practitioners advise regular, systematic meditation to create health, treat disease, and become rejuvenated. Set up a schedule to do the meditations in this book. Meditate on a mandala or another image of significance to you. Chant a mantra or pray.

Critically analyze your thoughts. Uncover what bothers you. Let go of negativity. Make amends for your wrongdoing. Start with amends to yourself. Heal your troubled relationships and cultivate healthy friendships. To avoid being abused, set appropriate boundaries. Transform dissonance into harmony in your mind and life.

Remember your dreams and figure out their meaning. Dreams shed light on what is going on in your mind and life. Wisdom dreams during the early morning *loong* period offer guidance.

Behave ethically, regardless of how other people treat you. Practice self-compassion and universal compassion. Take every opportunity to help others. Do what you enjoy. Create meaning from challenging situations and evolve to a higher state of consciousness.

MEDICINES

Composites

Practitioners prescribe medicines, based on complex Tibetan pharmaceutical formulae, if diet and behavior don't heal imbalance. Tibetan medicines are composites of medicinal plants. Some medicines have more than one hundred ingredients. The various components work together to reverse the underlying imbalance, treat the disorder's symptoms, heal any side effects from the medicines, and strengthen the body.

Compared with Western pharmaceuticals, Tibetan medicines are organic and gentle, with minimal side effects. They work slowly, except for some medicinal components that treat fever, inflammatory pain, indigestion, food poisoning, and other acute conditions. In the United States, they are categorized as food supplements.

Tibetan medical students at qualified Tibetan medical colleges go on regular field trips during which they learn to identify and pick medicinal plants, often growing high in the Himalayas. They transport the plants back to their medical college pharmacies for processing into medicines. The best medical college pharmacies use modern technology, sanitation, and quality control. Excellent pharmacies follow the essence of the guidelines explained in the *Gyueshi* and other Tibetan medical texts.

A few Tibetan medicines contain minute amounts of minerals, such as detoxified mercury. According to the *Gyueshi*, mercury is the king of poison, but detoxified mercury is the king of medicine. Ancient Tibetan medicine practitioners created a complex process to detoxify mercury and enhance the medicine's therapeutic value.

Tibetan medicines have four characteristics: taste, post-digestive taste, potency, and method of combining ingredients. This information is derived from the initial taste, taste after digestion, active ingredients, qualities, scent, color, and form. Plants with similar taste, potency, and post-digestive taste are compounded together.

Tibetan medicines are administered in various forms: decoction, broth, powder, general pills, precious pills, paste, syrup, medicinal butter, and medicinal wine. Practitioners prescribe the form that best treats the disorder. Tibetan pills come in assorted sizes ranging from hard to semi-hard. Crush a pill with mortar and pestle or dissolve it in a small cup of boiled water. Then swallow the crushed/softened pill, followed by a cup of boiled water, cooled enough to drink.

Right Medicine, at the Right Time, in the Right Way

Practitioners prescribe Tibetan medicines according to the disorder's manifesting time of day, the person's dietary habits, and nature of the imbalance. Tibetan medicines are dispensed in ten ways: early in the morning on an empty stomach, between meals, just before a meal, with a meal, just after a meal, after digestion of a meal, frequent small doses, mixed with food, both right before and right after a meal, and before bed.

Tibetan medicine advocates gentle treatment. Practitioners proceed carefully by prescribing a small dose on a trial basis. Baby steps can keep the medicine and affected primary energy from creating dysfunction in the other *nyepa*. For example, a proper medicine warms **loong** and **baekan** without aggravating **tripa**. Practitioners may increase the dose after developing better understanding of the disorder. If a larger dose doesn't reverse the imbalance, other Tibetan medicines may be prescribed.

Practitioners must prescribe each medicine correctly. Moreover, the medicine must be taken as directed. Prescribing and/or taking the wrong medicine, in the wrong way, at the wrong time may generate a new disorder without treating the initial one.

If a practitioner prescribes Tibetan medicines for you, tell her or him if you are using any other medicines, pharmaceuticals, and/or food supplements. Ask where the Tibetan medicines came from, what their purpose is, when to take them, and what side effects may occur. Make sure that the medicines were made by qualified Tibetan medical pharmacies. Tell your other health professionals that you are taking Tibetan medicines.

Cooling, Warming, or Neutral

Practitioners categorize Tibetan medicines according to whether they reverse hot disorders or cold disorders, or if they are neutral. They prescribe warming medicines for **loong** and/or **baekan** imbalance. Medicines with cooling qualities treat **tripa** imbalance. Warm, nutritious medicines are therapeutic for combined disorders of **loong** and **baekan**. Cool medicines treat combined disorders of **loong** and **tripa**. Cool, light medicines are remedies for combined disorders of **tripa** and **baekan**.

Pacification or Evacuation

Some Tibetan medicines pacify an imbalance. When a disorder is in a state of accumulation, practitioners prescribe a pacifying medicine. Pacification can be cool or warm, and the medicines may be a decoction, power, pill, paste, medicinal butter, or medicinal wine. Generally, medicinal butter and medicinal wine pacify **loong**, decoctions and powders pacify **tripa**, and pills and calcinated powders pacify **baekan**.

Other Tibetan medicines evacuate an imbalance. Evacuation medicines range from mild to strong. These medicines are administered as enemas, laxatives, emetics, and nasal cleansing. For example, vomiting evacuates *baekan* disorders located in the site of undigested food. Enemas expel *tripa* disorders in the site of digested food.

Pacification and evacuation complement each other. For example, medicines that increase digestive heat pacify indigestion. After symptoms decrease, practitioners prescribe medicines to evacuate the disorder from the passage closest to its location.

Pacification and evacuation work together to produce needed weight loss. Proper weight has many benefits: clearer sense organs, a feeling of lightness, appropriate appetite, smooth bowel movements, and balanced *loong* energy. To lose weight, practitioners recommend warming *baekan*. If evacuation is needed, practitioners may prescribe mild enemas.

However, excessive slimming therapy depletes the body constituents and increases susceptibility to contagious diseases, nausea, and *loong* disorders. Losing too much weight too fast leads to emaciation, poor complexion, giddiness, insomnia, thirst, loss of appetite, and weakening of the voice and sensory functions. Pain and disturbance may develop in the calves, thighs, coccyx, ribs, heart, and brain. Weight loss needs to be appropriate to support health.

Tibetan Precious Pills

Tibetan Precious Pills are the most powerful, deep-acting Tibetan medicines. Harvesting medicinal plants, purifying them, and combining the ingredients is done according to ancient Tibetan formulas. These sacred pills are composed of plants and minute amounts of powder derived from detoxified minerals. During each stage from harvest through administration, Tibetan Precious Pills are consecrated to maximize benefits.

Practitioners prescribe Tibetan Precious Pills for prevention and treatment of illness, as well as for rejuvenation. The pills produce a healthy complexion and they clear the sensory organs. They strengthen bones, open body channels, and increase vitality.

Ingesting a Tibetan Precious Pill is best done under the supervision of a Tibetan medicine practitioner. Except in an emergency, take this sacred pill on a full or new moon day. Ideally, ingest the pill on an auspicious date and at a time that a Tibetan astrologer forecasts.

The night prior to taking a Tibetan Precious Pill, drink pure, boiled water, cooled enough to drink. This water will open your body channels. Open the package and put the pill into a clean cup, without exposing it to light. Add a small amount of pure, boiled, hot water. Cover the cup with a clean lid and let the cup stand overnight.

Early the next morning, prepare yourself spiritually for ingesting the Tibetan Precious Pill. Chant the Medicine Buddha Mantra, while visualizing the pill healing you completely (see chapter 7). Then chant the mantra *Om Mani Padme Hum* as you let go of the three mental poisons and flood your entire self with compassion and wisdom (see chapter 5).

Stir the pill mixture in the cup and drink the contents. Then drink a cup of pure, boiled, slightly cooled water. Go to bed and cover yourself with warm bedding. After 15–30 minutes, get out of bed. Drink another cup of pure, boiled, slightly cooled water.

For the next couple of days, take it easy so that the Tibetan Precious Pill works. Avoid eating raw vegetables and fruits, fish, pork, eggs, sour drinks, alcohol, garlic, onion, rancid foods, and spicy foods that can cause indigestion. Refrain from strenuous exercise and sexual intercourse. Continue visualizing the Tibetan Precious Pill healing you completely.

ACCESSORY THERAPIES

Practitioners administer accessory treatments if diet, behavior, and medicines don't heal symptoms and the underlying imbalance. Accessory therapies are external interventions to pacify and evacuate disorders. Only qualified, experienced practitioners should administer them. Accessory therapies are divided into two categories: mild and strong.

Mild Accessory Therapies

- **Compress**: Place a pad of absorbent material onto a body part. A cold compress can relieve inflammation, decrease pain, and stop bleeding. A warm compress can decrease pain, increase circulation, and/or provide heat.

- **Hydrotherapy**: Take a medicinal bath or a shower; immerse the body in cool water, hot springs, or mineral waters to cool *tripa* or warm *loong* and *baekan*.
- **Massage**: Manually manipulate the soft body tissues (muscle, connective tissue, tendons, ligaments) to promote relaxation, circulation, and well-being.
- **Aromatherapy**: Breathe in or apply on the body essential oils to relax, enhance digestion, and relieve pain and nausea.

Strong Accessory Therapies

- **Acupressure**: Press pressure points to stimulate natural healing.
- **Venesection** (phlebotomy): Make an incision in a vein to withdraw blood and relieve a hot imbalance.
- **Moxibustion**: Burn a *moxa* on a specific point to stimulate the flow of energy, get rid of toxins, and reverse a cold disorder.
- **Golden-needle therapy**: Insert a warm needle in the Crown Chakra (*chee-tsuk*) on top of the head, put a *moxa* on the needle's upper tip, and burn the *moxa* to treat a cold dysfunction.
- **Cupping**: Insert fire into a copper cup to remove oxygen and create a vacuum; put the cup opening over a painful area to heat pores, stimulate energy and blood flow, break up obstructions, and pull out toxins.
- **Steam bath**: Use steam to raise the body temperature and treat a cold disorder.

Use of Accessory Therapies to Treat Imbalances

- **Treat *loong* disorders** with gentle, warming oil massages; hot, salty compresses on painful areas; and mild enemas to warm cold dysfunction and evacuate toxins.
- **Treat *tripa* disorders** with cooling medicinal oil massages, venesection, and cleansing to evacuate hot dysfunction.
- **Treat *baekan* disorders** with emesis to evacuate digestive dysfunction, as well as warm medicinal baths and natural springs to treat skin rashes, chronic arthritis, gout, rheumatism, and stiffness of the extremities resulting from cold imbalance.

PROGNOSIS

Good Prognosis

Practitioners determine prognosis to evaluate the effectiveness of the treatment. The prognosis is good for people who are young, courageous, and previously healthy. They honestly reply to practitioners' inquiries. Asking insightful questions, they work with practitioners to understand the dysfunction and how to heal it.

Individuals have a good prognosis if they make appropriate dietary and behavioral changes and use Tibetan medicines and accessory therapies as prescribed. They have resources to access appropriate treatment, and they tolerate this treatment. Their caregivers are trustworthy, loving, capable, compassionate, clean, and intelligent. These conditions promote recovery.

The nature of the imbalance affects prognosis. Easily cured disorders have insignificant causes, manifestations, and symptoms. Prognosis is good for people whose constitution doesn't have the same nature as the imbalance. For example, they have a *tripa* constitution and a *loong* or *baekan* imbalance. They are likely to recover if complications don't occur and only one body passage and one primary energy are affected.

Poor Prognosis

Prognosis is poor for people whose life and dysfunction are complicated. They require many kinds of treatment, including long-term therapy but can't access the care they need. Prognosis is not good for individuals who detest themselves, their health-care providers, and everyone else. Rebellious, they don't follow the prescribed treatment. Because they are angry and depressed, they waste their precious energy and exhaust their life span.

No remedies heal all disorders. Despite proper treatment, imbalance may result in fatal disease. Exceptional practitioners honestly explain the trajectory of the illness and when death is likely to occur. By learning their prognosis, individuals can put their affairs in order and create a good death, as explained in chapter 9.

MEDITATION ON SOUND

For millennia, sound has been used for meditation and healing. Ancient sages learned that naturally occurring, vibrating sounds promote physical, mental, and spiritual health. Some traditions teach that music is based on celestial sounds experienced during deep meditation. Tibetans play singing bowls and musical instruments as part of meditation.

Om (*A-U-M*) is said to be the primordial sound from which all creation arises. *Om Mani Padme Hum* and many other Sanskrit mantras begin with *Om*. The sound of *Om* has four unique parts: (1) *Ah*, (2) *Uh*, (3) *Mmm*, and (4) silence. Each sound vibrates in a different part of the body. On the internet you can listen to the sound of *Om* (*A-U-M*). Chant *Om* (*A-U-M*) or meditate on another sound, such as ocean waves, to calm, heal, and revitalize yourself.

How to Meditate on Sound

- Sit comfortably in a straight-back chair, a meditation cushion, or on the floor; or lie on the bed with your arms along your sides.
- Straighten your back and breathe deeply.
- Lower or close your eyes, relax your entire body, and mentally push away all distractions.
- Breathe in a circular manner, through your nostrils, from your abdomen, slowly, deeply, evenly, with your in-breath the same length as your out-breath, and no break in between; keep breathing in this manner throughout and after the meditation.
- Chant (*A-U-M*) on a note that is comfortable; hear and feel the vibration in your body.
- Meditate on the silence between each sound; let the sounds take you to a deeper level and learn what is in your unconscious mind.
- After completing your meditation, open your eyes fully and take into your everyday life your insight from this meditation.

You can use Sound Meditation to focus on a pleasant sound, such as beautiful music. Sound Meditation will help you to cope with annoying noises like building construction and people talking on cell phones.

Meditate on the sound, rather than get upset with the din. You will transform the hubbub into peace and insight.

This chapter addressed how Tibetan medicine practitioners create individualized treatment plans. After identifying the treatment goal, they prescribe four levels of therapy. First, they recommend a healthy diet and behavior. If these changes don't reverse imbalance, they prescribe medicines and accessory therapies. They evaluate the effectiveness of treatment by determining the prognosis. The chapter ends with Meditation on Sound to reverse imbalance and promote peace.

Chapters 1–9 explained how to use Tibetan medicine as self-care. Chapters 10–14 described Tibetan medicine from the point of view of Tibetan medicine practitioners. These two perspectives will help you to use Tibetan medicine for your self-care and integrative care plan.

If you are a health professional working in conventional care, you may wonder about the scientific basis of Tibetan medicine. The last chapter, chapter 15, reviews the latest relevant, published studies in scientific journals. You will learn how to practice research-based self-care and integrative care that includes Tibetan medicine.

• 15 •

Tibetan Medicine for Health Professionals

$\mathcal{C}$onventional health care, often called modern medicine or Western medicine, has made impressive strides to treat illness. However, much of the health-care dollar is spent on caring for people whose chronic health problems result, in part, from their unhealthy lifestyle choices. Even individuals with access to affordable conventional care may not find the help they need to create health, recover from disease, and deal well with death. That's why many people are looking outside of conventional care for cost-effective answers to better health.

In the United States, more than 30 percent of adults and approximately 12 percent of children use complementary and alternative therapies. Complementary therapies are nonmainstream practices integrated into conventional care, whereas alternative therapies are nonmainstream practices used in place of conventional care.[1] Integrating complementary therapies into conventional care promotes empowerment and offers more options than using only one type of care. Tibetan medicine, Tibet's ancient science of healing, is a timely, cost-effective complementary therapy for self-care and integrative care.

Often, nonconventional complementary therapies lack scientific evidence. The scientific method doesn't easily adapt to investigating traditional holistic healing systems. Even so, publications are exploding with studies about the benefits of interventions integral to Tibetan medicine. This ancient tradition and, increasingly, conventional care share the perspective that everyone is born with unique, interrelated mental, physical, and spiritual needs. Tibetan medicine offers a model for inexpensive self-care and integrative care that complements conventional care.

If you are a health professional working in conventional health care, you may wonder how to use Tibetan medicine for your own self-care and as part of integrative care. This chapter explains what you can do. For details, see the previous fourteen chapters. This chapter gives an overview of Tibetan medicine pertinent to conventional health professionals, examines the scientific basis, and explains application and effectiveness. In conclusion, the chapter describes the meditation at the heart of Tibetan medicine: *Loving-Kindness Is My Religion*. Using Tibetan medicine for self-care and integrative care promotes relationship-based, individualized, quality care.

OVERVIEW FOR HEALTH PROFESSIONALS

Background

The earliest inhabitants of Tibet learned to thrive in the Himalayas, the tallest mountains on earth. Observing wildlife, ancient Tibetans relied on natural resources to heal and sustain them. They practiced *Bon*, Tibet's indigenous shamanism, based on the interrelatedness of mind, body, and the natural world. When Buddhism came to Tibet, Tibetan medicine evolved into a blend of *Bon* and Buddhism, with influences from yoga and Ayurveda in India and traditional medicine in China, Persia, and Greece. In the eighth century, Yuthok Yonten Gonpo, a famous doctor of Tibetan medicine, compiled these teachings into the *Gyueshi*, the fundamental text of Tibetan medicine.

Today, the best Tibetan medical colleges base their programs on the *Gyueshi*, commentaries, research, experience, and current theories of health and disease. For example, students at the Men-Tsee-Khang Medical College in Dharamsala, India, study the *Gyueshi* during a five-year program plus an internship of one or two years. Graduates become a doctor of Tibetan medicine, called a Tibetan medicine practitioner in the United States. After ten years of practice, they are eligible to take an exam to earn the distinguished *Men-Rampa* degree.

Also, Tibetan medical students study the *Gyueshi* at the Tibetan Medical College, Tso-Ngon (Qinghai) University in Amdo on the Tibetan Plateau. Medical students can earn a bachelor's degree, master's degree, and PhD in Tibetan medicine. Nursing students earn a bachelor's degree in Tibetan medicine nursing. Nursing graduates take the same licensing exam as other nurses on the Tibetan Plateau.

Karma, Suffering, Healing, and Happiness

Tibetan medicine is based on four profound teachings: karma, suffering, healing, and happiness. Karma is the universal law of cause and effect, "As you sow, so will you reap." Creating health and happiness requires good choices. Ethical behavior is essential to avoid turmoil. Sometimes choices have immediate results. Other times, effects are not readily apparent. For example, eating an unhealthy diet and living an inappropriate lifestyle may not reap poor consequences immediately but eventually will cause suffering and dis-ease (lack of ease). Mindfulness is needed to recognize immediate and long-term effects of choices.

Suffering results from interpreting situations negatively. The Sanskrit term for suffering is *dukkha* or dis-satisfaction (lack of satisfaction). Most of human life is spent trying to avoid suffering and increase pleasure, often in ways that inadvertently cause suffering. Pain and suffering aren't the same. For example, being angry about a broken leg intensifies the pain and causes suffering. Anger makes things worse.

Healing means to reestablish balance and create optimal health. Purify negativity and behave ethically. A compassionate, positive mindset promotes clear thinking and healthy choices that maintain balance. The mind can heal, even as the body is dying.

Happiness is the very purpose of life. Happiness results from a peaceful mind and balanced life. To create meaning, reach out to help others and see your life as part of a bigger, purposeful picture. Even in challenging circumstances, behave with integrity according to the highest ethical values. Like a lotus flower growing in a swamp, you can transform life's "mud" into nourishment to rise and bloom.

Energy: The Source of Existence

All phenomena are a manifestation of *joong-wa-nya*, the Tibetan term for the five sources of energy. Translated as five elements, they are **earth**, **water**, **fire**, **air**, and **space**. Ancient Tibetans used everyday terms to illustrate their universal, energetic qualities. The five elements consist of physiologic functions that work synergistically to maintain physical, mental, and spiritual health (see chapter 3). You are connected to everyone and everything because of *nue-pa*, the Tibetan word for energy.

The five elements interact to form three primary energies, called *nyepa* in Tibetan, that are essential for life. Each *nyepa* has divisions, subdivisions, and defining characteristics. **Loong**, movement energy, is pronounced loong. **Loong** promotes creativity and spirituality. **Tripa**, heat energy, is pronounced teepa. **Tripa** is essential for metabolic, endocrine functions and for setting and meeting goals. **Baekan**, cold energy, is pronounced bacon. **Baekan** provides grounding, moisture, and tolerance.

You, like everyone else, were born with a unique combination of *nyepa*, called your constitution. Your dominant energy or energies give the name to your constitution. You have characteristics of all three energies. However, your dominant energy or energies exert the greatest influence. If, for example, you have a **tripa/baekan** constitution, **tripa** and **baekan** influence you more than **loong** does.

Ordinarily, your inborn constitution doesn't change. However, countless variables cause your *nyepa* to rise, fall, and/or become disturbed. Examples are your thoughts, diet, behavior, work, stress, weather, environment, other people, time of day, and stage in life. You create health and happiness by making choices that keep the current percentages of your **loong**, **tripa**, and **baekan** about the same as their percentages in your constitution. Learning about your constitution will help you to maintain balance.

Health = Balance and Disease = Imbalance

Suffering and dis-ease (lack of ease) begin in the mind. Thoughts impact the *nyepa*. Happiness helps to balance **loong**, **tripa**, and **baekan** and enhance immunity. In contrast, negative thinking, called mental poisons, promotes poor choices that lead to imbalance, suffering, and illness.

For example, anger increases the heart rate and blood pressure, and depresses the immune system. Anger causes shallow, irregular breathing that fails to oxygenate the cells properly and get rid of toxins. Rather than becoming angry, you can transform this negativity into compassion. Then you will think more clearly about how to deal with the situation in a manner that creates good consequences.

Tibetan medicine describes three categories of mental poisons that are disastrous for mind and body. These mental poisons are (1) greed, attachment, and desire; (2) anger, hostility, and aggression; and (3) delusion, confusion, and closed-mindedness. This negativity causes *loong*, *tripa*, and *baekan* to go out of balance and create health problems.

Your constitution makes you susceptible to specific mental poisons and related health problems. A *loong* constitution makes you vulnerable to engaging in greed, attachment, and desire. In other words, greed causes and results from *loong* imbalance. This imbalance can produce anxiety, lack of focus, movement disorders, insomnia, mental illness, and addictions.

If you have a *tripa* constitution, you are prone to engaging in anger, hostility, and aggression. Anger causes and results from *tripa* imbalance. Too much, too little, or disturbed heat can lead to inflammations, infections, skin eruptions, metabolic and hormonal dysfunction, and emotional and physical violence.

Likewise, a *baekan* constitution makes you susceptible to engaging in delusion, confusion, and closed-mindedness. Delusion causes and results from *baekan* imbalance. To much, too little, or disturbed cold can produce respiratory disorders, obesity, diabetes, lethargy, and dementia.

A dual constitution gives ready access to both dominant energies. However, you also are prone to the mental poisons of both dominant *nyepa*. If, for example, you have a *loong/tripa* constitution, you are susceptible to greed and anger.

When one *nyepa* goes out of balance, the other two primary energies are likely to go out of balance, too. Anxiety and insomnia often begin the process. *Loong* rises too high, which affects *tripa* and *baekan*. Chronic imbalance in all three *nyepa* is difficult to unravel and can produce complex health problems, such as auto-immune disorders, diabetes, and cardiovascular disease. By making good choices, you heal your mind, whether or not your body is cured, and transform suffering into happiness.

SCIENTIFIC BASIS

Traditional Research

Tibetan medicine is based on observations and theories of the mind-body-natural world connection. Since ancient times, Tibetan medicine practitioners have conducted research to practice evidence-based medicine. After documenting results, they prescribed the most effective treatments. They passed down this information to Tibetan medical students and practitioners from one generation to the next. Now scientific researchers are validating many of these health claims.

Tibetan Medicine as a Holistic System

Scientific studies report positive findings about Tibetan medicine as a holistic system.[2] Tibetan medicine had beneficial effects on quality of life, disease regression, and remission in persons with cancer and blood disorders.[3] Women with breast cancer who did Tibetan yoga during chemotherapy showed improved sleep quality.[4] Anthropological studies have produced qualitative interpretations of Tibetan medical theories and practices.[5, 6, 7, 8, 9, 10]

Cameron et al.[11] tested and refined two self-assessment tools based on Tibetan medicine as a holistic system: (1) Constitutional Self-Assessment Tool (CSAT) and (2) Lifestyle Guidelines Tool (LGT). As stated in chapter 2, both tools had high content validity. The CSAT had moderate criterion validity, which increased for participants who knew the basic teachings of Tibetan medicine and did accurate self-assessments.

Healing Practices Integral to Tibetan Medicine

For millennia, Tibetan medicine has advocated healing practices. Numerous studies have found benefits from interventions that are essential to Tibetan medicine. Examples are acupressure, aromatherapy, breathing techniques, imagery, listening, presence, and therapeutic touch.[12] Research findings are positive for art therapy,[13] meditation,[14] and mindfulness.[15] Moreover, music therapy, reflexology, Reiki,[16] and yoga[17] demonstrate usefulness in multiple health situations. Increasingly, these ancient, inexpensive therapies are becoming a popular part of conventional care.

Compassion

Compassion, the essence of Tibetan medicine, is a philosophical stance of kindness toward all individuals, regardless of how they behave. Rather than a feeling, compassion is an understanding that all phenomena are made of the same five energy sources. Fernando, Rea, and Malpas[18] found that compassion consists of connection, presence, warmth, respect, and caring. Tibetan medicine advocates these compassion practices.

Tibetan medicine teaches a positive relationship between self-compassion, universal compassion, health, and happiness. Numerous studies have confirmed this connection. Researchers have found this relationship in a variety of individuals including adolescents and adults,[19] nurses,[20] children,[21] and postpartum women at risk for depression and anxiety.[22]

Many researchers have studied so-called compassion fatigue. According to Tibetan medicine, compassion fatigue doesn't exist because compassion doesn't cause exhaustion. Rather, compassion fatigue is codependency, defined as enabling addiction, poor mental health, and irresponsibility. Codependents feel burned out, go beyond their personal limits, and need other people's approval. In studies of nurses, these characteristics were inversely related to self-compassion.[23]

Papadopoulos et al.[24] found that nurses in fifteen countries agreed about the importance and attributes of compassion. Wishing to provide compassionate care was insufficient, though, without cultivation of compassion[25] and a supportive work setting.[26] In a study by Barron, Deery, and Sloan,[27] mental health nurses needed encouragement to develop self-compassion and work toward a greater understanding of compassionate care.

Health professionals will benefit from Tibetan medicine's perspective on compassion. They will develop a deeper understanding of compassion. This knowledge will empower them to practice self-compassion and deliver compassionate care. Educators of health professionals will teach compassion. Researchers will conduct more studies about compassion.

Tibetan Medicines

Most published research about Tibetan medicine focuses on the efficacy of Tibetan medicines. Conducting this research is challenging. Each Tibetan medicine consists of multiple herbal ingredients to treat symptoms, reverse imbalance, and promote healing with minimal side-effects.[28] Testing each ingredient in a Tibetan medicine is complicated and expensive. Medicinal plants do not have the same uniformity as pharmaceuticals.[29]

Even so, research results are promising. Namdul et al.[30] found that Tibetan medicines had a significant positive effect on persons with type 2 diabetes. *Liucha* (young leaves and shoots of *Sibiraea laevigata*) showed more potent alpha-glucosidase inhibitory activity than the drug *acarbose*.[31] Tibetan medicines reduced symptoms of multiple sclerosis.[32] *Padma 28*, a Tibetan medicine, lessened pain and increased walking distance in persons with intermittent claudication.[33] Feng et al.[34] found that the fruit and leaf of *Vaccinium Glaucoalbum* had strong antioxidant activity. Tibetan turnip promoted hypoxia tolerance in healthy humans.[35]

Currently, most studies using Tibetan medicines are being conducted on rats and mice in laboratories. Recent findings indicated anti-tumor activity,[36] lower uric acid,[37] decreased MCF7 breast cancer cells,[38] and reduced neuropathic pain.[39] *Tsantan Sumtang*, a Tibetan medicine, targeted and regulated multiple perturbed pathways in cardiopyretic disease.[40]

Future Research

Additional high-quality, evidence-based studies are needed about Tibetan medicines. For example, researchers could investigate little-understood active ingredients. Unknowns hamper establishment of drug quality standards, development of new medicines, commercial production of medicines, and marketing of medicines. Research will help outdated Tibetan pharmacies to modernize, verify clinical efficacy, and write criteria to guide clinical practice.

Currently, Tibetan medicines aren't readily accessible for non-Tibetans. Research can determine if Tibetan medicines would benefit the larger community. If so, studies can investigate if and how to make quality Tibetan medicines available more widely. Ethical issues must be addressed about safeguarding each medicine's recipe, or pharmaceutical companies may use the recipe to make money, without fair reimbursement to the Tibetan community.

Research is needed to examine Tibetan medicine as a holistic system. Conducting this research is challenging. The profound practices affect mind and body in ways that are not reproducible and quantifiable. If studies don't investigate the same variables, findings are difficult to com-

pare. Most published research was conducted for a brief time. Longitu-
dinal studies are crucial to understand long-term effects. New qualitative
methods may be needed to investigate Tibetan medicine's synergistic
interplay of physical, mental, ethical, and spiritual components.

Studies are needed to understand how Tibetan medicine practitioners and other health professionals view integrative care that includes
Tibetan medicine and conventional care. The findings will offer insight
into issues that must be addressed in order for these professionals to
collaborate without usurping and taking credit for each other's expertise. Successfully tackling such challenges is essential to provide quality
integrative care.

Tibetan medicine generates many research questions. Investigating these and other questions will guide the use of Tibetan medicine for
self-care and integrative care:

- Why is mind integral to health, happiness, and disease?
- How does Tibetan medicine as a holistic approach affect happiness, health, disease, immunity, longevity, rejuvenation, and
  preparation for death?
- What are the relationships between each of Tibetan medicine's
  seven general constitutions and measurements of anxiety, insomnia, anger, depression, addictions, and biological markers?
- To what extent is Tibetan medicine correct about the three
  nyepa, seven constitutions, and relationships between energy
  imbalance and specific health problems?
- To what degree is Tibetan pulse diagnosis reliable and valid?
- How can health professionals promote Tibetan medicine for
  self-care and integrative care?
- Can Tibetan medicinal herbs from the Himalayas be grown at
  sea level in the Western Hemisphere? If so, do these herbs have
  the same potency as those harvested in the Himalayas?
- Are Tibetan medicines that contain detoxified mercury and
  other heavy metals safe?
- Which Tibetan medicines are effective for treating which health
  problems?
- Does an individual's constitution affect the efficacy of a Tibetan
  medicine?

APPLICATION

Ideally, Tibetan medicine practitioners and conventional health practitioners work side by side as partners to provide quality integrative care. They avoid infringing on each other's scope of practice and jeopardizing care. Conventional health professionals who try to practice Tibetan medicine run the risk of appropriating this ancient science of healing without giving proper recognition to and truly understanding Tibetan medicine, and vice versa for Tibetan medicine practitioners. If so, they devalue each other's discipline while co-opting the practices. Infrastructures are needed that promote effective, egalitarian communication and collaboration between Tibetan medicine practitioners and other health professionals.

The next sections give practical suggestions for how you, a health professional in conventional care, can use Tibetan medicine for self-care and integrative care. You can benefit from Tibetan medicine without encroaching on the professional practice of Tibetan medicine practitioners and going beyond your scope of practice. Besides applying these practices in your own life, you can share them, as appropriate, with individuals for whom you provide care. Tibetan medicine can help you to evolve into a true healer.

Live in Harmony with Your Inborn Constitution

To create health and happiness, you need to live in harmony with your constitution. The gold standard for constitutional analysis is a consultation with an experienced, qualified practitioner of Tibetan medicine. The practitioner observes you, analyzes your urine, reads your radial pulses, and questions you. Using this information, the practitioner assesses your constitution, what if any *nyepa* are out of balance, and how to bring them back into balance. The practitioner recommends supportive lifestyle choices, as explained in chapter 13.

Before a consultation, complete the Constitutional Self-Assessment Tool (CSAT). To increase the accuracy of your CSAT result, read the basic teachings of Tibetan medicine, as explained in this book, and follow the instructions in chapter 2. Use your CSAT result to complete the Lifestyle Guidelines Tool (LGT). Create a plan for living in harmony with your constitution. The CSAT and LGT are posted online for anyone to complete anonymously for free, 24/7.[41]

Create a Healthy Mind

When engaging in negativity, you are likely to make poor lifestyle choices that undermine you. A clear mind helps you to choose what leads to health and happiness. Create a healthy mind by transforming the three kinds of mental poisons into positive behavior, as described in table 15.1.

Table 15.1. How to Heal the Three Mental Poisons

Mental poison	Causes imbalance in	Meditate on	Action
Greed, attachment, desire	**Loong**	Impermanence: continuous change	Generosity, acceptance
Anger, hostility, aggression	**Tripa**	Yearn for everyone to be free of suffering	Reach out and ask, "How can I help?"
Delusion, confusion, closed-mindedness	**Baekan**	Wisdom: Wake up!	Cultivate mindfulness of the moment

Tibetan medicine integrates ethics, spirituality, and healing. Root out negativity and live an ethical, spiritual life. Happiness results from behaving with compassion, love, kindness, contentment, honesty, integrity, forgiveness, joy, peace, tolerance, meaning, altruism, humility, responsibility, equanimity, and patience. Chapters 8 and 9 explain how to create a healthy, enlightened mind.

Meditation is a powerful intervention to cultivate optimal health and a happy mind. As numerous studies have found, meditation opens the heart, promotes compassion, and enhances the immune system.[42] During meditation, the mind may seem like a jumping monkey, leaping from thought to thought. Tibetan meditation tames the monkey mind.

In Tibetan medicine, the overall purpose of meditation is to become familiar with and purify the mind. This process involves bringing unconscious thoughts into the conscious mind to heal negativity. Many options exist: Meditate while sitting, walking, lying down, dancing, and/or listening to calming music. Exercising first may promote quiet during sitting meditation. The ideal is to develop a meditative perspective all the time.

You can start with a two-minute meditation on your breath every couple of hours. Before getting out of bed, meditate for two minutes. Stop to meditate before leaving your car and buying groceries. From short meditations, move on to other meditations in this book.

How to Do a Two-Minute Meditation on Your Breath

- Make yourself comfortable sitting, standing, walking, or lying down.
- Straighten your back, relax your body, lower or close your eyes, and breathe deeply.
- Engage in circular breathing: Breathe slowly and deeply through your nose, from your abdomen, with your in-breath the same length as out-breath, and no break in between.
- Focus on your breath; feel the warmth of the out-breath and coolness of the in-breath.
- When your attention wanders, bring it gently back to your breath; counting your breaths can help you to focus.
- After completing your meditation, continue to engage in circular breathing.

The meditations in this book use circular breathing. Engaging in circular breathing all the time brings in life force, oxygenates the cells, and releases toxins. You can do these meditations at home, use them at work, and teach them to people for whom you provide care. Circular breathing and meditation before, during, and after tests, treatments, and surgery calms mind and body.

Create a Healthy Body

The CSAT identifies your current dominant energy that may not be the same as the dominant energy in your inborn constitution if an imbalance exists. Using your CSAT result, follow the LGT column to calm **loong**, cool **tripa**, or warm **baekan**. If, for example, your CSAT result is **loong**, use the **loong** column to calm **loong**. Periodically completing the CSAT and LGT together will help you to bring the current percentages of your *nyepa* into balance and keep them in sync with your constitution.

Diet and behavior are the most important therapies. Ingest foods and beverages and engage in behaviors that support your constitution. In chapter 2, the LGT lists optimal food and behavior for *loong, tripa,* and *baekan.* You can bring your *nyepa* into balance by eating food and doing what is opposite to your CSAT dominant energy. Chapter 8 explains how to create a healthy body.

When stressed-out and *loong* is high, calm *loong* by doing what is grounded, peaceful, and warm. Ingest warm, nutritious food, such as soup, and sit quietly. On a scorching day when *tripa* is elevated, cool *tripa* by doing what is dry and cool. Eat cool, fresh salads, and stay out of the hot sun. During a frigid winter when *baekan* rises, warm *baekan* by doing what is dry and warm. Ingest a warm, spicy diet and exercise vigorously.

Create a healthy body and mind by spending time safely in nature. Because you are part of nature, being in nature is restorative, as many studies affirm.[43] For example, forest bathing reduced symptoms in elders with chronic heart failure.[44] Meditate while you are walking safely in a beautiful setting. If you can't immerse yourself in nature, meditate on a photo of a lotus flower, a lake, a waterfall, or the ocean. Even viewing videos of beautiful landscapes can produce physiological and psychological relaxation.[45]

How to Meditate in Nature

- Walk or sit safely in a forest or nature center, by a lake or stream, in a garden, along the ocean, or in another beautiful area.
- Engage in circular breathing: Breathe slowly, deeply, evenly through your nose, from your abdomen, with your in-breath the same length as the out-breath, and no break in between.
- Look at the trees, flowers, water, birds, and other wildlife. Notice what color they are, what sounds they make, what their forms are, and what they are doing.
- Let go of your worries and immerse yourself in nature.
- Feel the joy of breathing in and out and being part of this picturesque scene.

Create a Good Death

Tibetan medicine teaches that death is part of life. You die like you live. To die well, you must live well. Negativity that you don't heal during life likely will cause suffering while you die.

Because you don't know when you will die, you are best off preparing for death now. Root out negativity and behave virtuously. Make amends for hurting yourself and others. Create a healthy, enlightened mind and meaningful life. Cultivate compassion and wisdom that help you to face death with acceptance, peace, and even joy. Chapter 9 explains how to create a good death and to provide physical, emotional, and spiritual support for someone who is dying.

EFFECTIVENESS

Gradual Change

To assess Tibetan medicine's effectiveness, determine if you feel better by applying these practices. Ask recipients of your care if the therapies are helpful for them. Conventional care may be best if pharmaceuticals, technology, and surgery are needed to treat acute illness or injury. Tibetan medicine can be effective to create a healthy mind and body, manage chronic illness, and die peacefully.

Tibetan medicine can help an individual with cancer to heal from chemotherapy and radiation that are treatments in conventional care. Someone with diabetes can follow the recommendations of conventional care and also use Tibetan medicine to create a balanced life and slow the onset of complications. Even beginners can use Tibetan medicine to decrease stress, anxiety, and headaches, and to improve digestion and sleep.

However, most health problems develop over time. Tibetan medicine may not heal them right away. Serious imbalance requires long-term rebalancing. Tibetan medicine calls for gradual change. Optimal benefits occur from systematic use.

Precautions

Precautions are needed to enhance the effectiveness of Tibetan medicine, conventional care, and any other healing system. Be mindful when integrating different approaches. Take informed steps to ensure coordinated, safe, quality care.

For example, don't use Tibetan medicine to replace effective conventional care or as a reason to postpone consulting with conventional health professionals, and vice versa. Learn as much as you can about your constitution and your health problems. Carefully select qualified experts you trust and with whom you have karmic links. Ask questions and advocate for yourself, rather than accept what experts say. Explain to these experts how you manage your health and medications you take. Consult with appropriate experts, but listen to your own internal wisdom.

Problems can occur when Tibetan medicine practitioners, as well as other health professionals, exceed their scope of practice. Because Tibetan medicine is new in the United States, standardization and accreditation have not yet been established. Some people who lack credentials claim to be Tibetan medicine practitioners. Only consult with experienced practitioners who graduated from a legitimate Tibetan medical college.

In the United States, Tibetan medicine practitioners must follow state laws regulating unlicensed practitioners of complementary and alternative health care. For example, chapter 146A of the 2018 Minnesota Statutes[46] states that unlicensed practitioners cannot call themselves a doctor or use treatments such as acupuncture, covered by other Minnesota state licensing boards. They must give each client a detailed bill of rights about their qualifications and the client's rights and responsibilities.

If practitioners prescribe Tibetan medicines, precautions are needed to ensure effective care. Tibetan medicines are composites of herbs picked primarily in the mountains. These preparations work slowly and gently and have few, if any, side effects. In the United States, Tibetan medicines are categorized as dietary supplements regulated by the Food and Drug Administration (FDA). In general, the regulations are less stringent than for pharmaceuticals.

A few Tibetan medicines contain minute amounts of minerals to enhance potency. In studies, Tibetan medicines containing detoxified mercury did not lead to mercury in the blood of human participants[47] and cause toxicity in human and rat liver cells or in zebrafish.[48] Researchers concluded that detoxified mercury did not have appreciable adverse effects and may have exerted a beneficial effect.[49] More studies are being conducted on detoxified mercury in Tibetan medicines. If you aren't satisfied with these studies, you easily can avoid taking Tibetan medicines that contain heavy metals.

If you are using pharmaceuticals, tell your Tibetan medicine practitioner before taking Tibetan medicines. Similarly, inform your conventional health professionals if you are taking Tibetan medicines. The actions of Tibetan medicines and pharmaceuticals may conflict with each other. Women who are pregnant or nursing and parents who want to use Tibetan medicines for children should first consult with qualified health professionals. Only take Tibetan medicines prescribed by experienced, qualified Tibetan medicine practitioners and made by qualified Tibetan medical pharmacies.

In summary, this chapter explained how conventional health professionals can use Tibetan medicine for self-care and integrative care. The chapter gave an overview of Tibetan medicine specific to health professionals and addressed the scientific basis, application, and effectiveness. Health professionals who use Tibetan medicine for self-care and integrative care will expand inexpensive, healing options and deliver research-based, individualized, quality care.

MEDITATION: LOVING-KINDNESS IS MY RELIGION

Tibetan medicine is a complex, holistic healing system based on Buddhist philosophy, psychology, and science of the mind. These profound teachings are beyond religion and can be understood on many levels. The essence of Tibetan medicine is to understand reality: the absence of an intrinsic self. The ultimate remedy for suffering and disease is to generate compassion and wisdom.

His Holiness the 14th Dalai Lama condensed Tibet's ancient, timely, life-transforming science of healing into one statement:

Loving-kindness is my religion.

Meditating on this affirmation purifies negativity and cultivates compassion and wisdom. Amid life's challenges, you behave ethically and evolve spiritually. Your life has meaning because you are part of a bigger, purposeful picture. You transform suffering into well-being, better health, and joy for yourself and others.

Notes

HIS HOLINESS THE 14TH DALAI LAMA MESSAGE

1. His Holiness the 14th Dalai Lama wrote this blessing for the work, including this book, of the Tibetan Healing Initiative, which is part of the Yoga and Tibetan Medicine Focus Area, led by Dr. Miriam E. Cameron, at the Earl E. Bakken Center for Spirituality & Healing, University of Minnesota. Retrieved from https://www.csh.umn.edu/education/focus-areas/tibetan-medicine/dalai-lama-blessing.

NOTES

1. Gonpo, Y. Y. (2015a). *Root Trantra and explanatory Tantra (Gyueshi)* (Trans., T. Paljor, P. Wangdu, & S. Dolma). Dharamsala, India: Men-Tsee-Khang.
2. Gonpo, Y. Y. (2015b). *Subsequent Tantra (Gyueshi)* (Trans., T. Paljor). Dharamsala, India: Men-Tsee-Khang.
3. Gonpo, Y. Y. (1888). *Gyueshi*. Lhasa: Chakpori Press.
4. Germano, D., & Tournadre, N. (2010). *THL simplified phonetic transcription of standard Tibetan*. Retrieved from http://www.thlib.org/reference/transliteration/#!essay=/thl/phonetics/s/b1.
5. Wylie, T. (1959). A standard system of Tibetan transcription. *Harvard Journal of Asiatic Studies, (22)*, 261–267.

INTRODUCTION

1. Cameron, M. E., Crisham, P., & Lewis, D. E. (1994). Content of ethical problems experienced by persons living with AIDS. *Journal of the Association of Nurses in AIDS Care, 5*(5), 32–42.
2. Cameron, M. E. (2002). Older persons' experience of ethical problems involving their health. *Nursing Ethics, 9*(5), 547–66.
3. Cameron, M. E., Schaffer, M., & Park, H. A. (2001). Nursing students' experience of ethical problems and use of ethical decision-making models. *Nursing Ethics, 8*(5), 432–47.
4. Park, H. A., Cameron, M. E., Han, S. S., Ahn, S. H., Oh, H. S., & Kim, K. U. (2003). Korean nursing students' ethical problems and ethical decision-making. *Nursing Ethics, 10*(6), 639–654.
5. Hammerschlag, C. A. (1988). *The dancing healers: A doctor's journey of healing with Native Americans.* New York: HarperOne, 45.
6. Cameron, M. E. (2002). *Karma & happiness: A Tibetan odyssey in ethics, spirituality, and healing.* Foreword by His Holiness the Dalai Lama. New York: Rowman & Littlefield.
7. Gonpo, Y. Y. (1888). *Gyueshi.* Lhasa: Chakpori Press.
8. Gonpo, Y. Y. (2015a). *Root Tantra and explanatory Tantra (Gyueshi)* (Trans., T. Paljor, P. Wangdu, & S. Dolma). Dharamsala, India: Men-Tsee-Khang.
9. Gonpo, Y. Y. (2015b). *Subsequent Tantra (Gyueshi)* (Trans., T. Paljor). Dharamsala, India: Men-Tsee-Khang.
10. Cameron, M. E. (1993). *Living with AIDS: Experiencing ethical problems* (Foreword, E. D. Pellegrino). Newbury Park, CA: Sage.
11. Cameron, M. E., Torkelson, C., Haddow, S., Namdul, T., Prasek, A., & Gross, C. (2012, May/June). Tibetan medicine and integrative health: Validity testing and refinement of the Constitutional Self-Assessment Tool and Lifestyle Guidelines Tool. *EXPLORE: The Journal of Science and Healing, 8*(3), 158–71.
12. Men-Tsee-Khang. (2017). *Fundamentals of Tibetan medicine.* Dharamsala, India: Author (back cover).

CHAPTER 2

1. Cameron, M. E. (1993). *Living with AIDS: Experiencing ethical problems* (Foreword, E. D. Pellegrino). Newbury Park, CA: Sage.

2. Cameron, M. E., Torkelson, C., Haddow, S., Namdul, T., Prasek, A., & Gross, C. R. (2012). Tibetan medicine and integrative health. *EXPLORE: The Journal of Science and Healing, 8*(3), 158–171.

3. Earl E. Bakken Center for Spirituality & Healing. (2019). *Constitutional Self-Assessment Tool (CSAT) and Lifestyle Guidelines Tool (LGT)*. Retrieved from https://www.csh.umn.edu/education/focus-areas/tibetan-medicine/assessment-and-guidelines-tools.

4. Earl E. Bakken Center for Spirituality & Healing. (2019). *CSPH 5315—Traditional Tibetan medicine: Ethics, spirituality, & healing*. Retrieved from https://www.csh.umn.edu/education/credit-courses/csph-5315-traditional-tibetan-medicine-ethics-spirituality-and-healing.

CHAPTER 3

1. Rinpoche, T. W. (2002). *Healing with form, energy and light* (Dahlby, M., Ed.). Ithaca, NY: Snow Lion Publications.

CHAPTER 6

1. Shantideva. (2003). *The way of the Bodhisattva* (Padmakara Translation Group, Trans.). Boston: Shambhala Classics.

2. Wallace, B. A., & Hodel, B. (2011). *Stilling the mind: Shamatha teachings from Dudjom Lingpa's Vajra Essence*. Somerville, MA: Wisdom Publications.

CHAPTER 9

1. Padmasambhava. (2005). *The Tibetan Book of the Dead: First complete translation*. Commentary by HH the Dalai Lama (revealed by T. K. Lingpa; G. Dorje; Ed.; G. Coleman with T. Jinpa, Trans.). New York: Penguin Books.

2. Evans-Wentz, W. Y. (1960). *The Tibetan Book of the Dead (The after-death experiences on the bardo plane, according to Lama Kazi Dawa-Samdup's English rendering)*. New York: Oxford University Press.

CHAPTER 10

1. Minnesota Legislature, Office of the Revisor of Statutes. (2018). *2018 Minnesota Statutes, Chapter 146A. Complementary and alternative health care practices.* Retrieved from https://www.revisor.mn.gov/statutes/cite/146A.

CHAPTER 15

1. Center for Complementary and Integrative Health (NCCIH, 2019). *Complementary, alternative, or integrative health.* Retrieved from https://nccih.nih.gov/health/integrative-health-types.

2. Cameron, M. E. (2018). Systems of care; Sowa Rigpa: The Tibetan knowledge of healing. In R. Lindquist, M. F. Tracy, & M. Snyder (Eds.), *Complementary/Alternative therapies in nursing* (8th Ed.) (chap. 5) (pp. 63–77). New York: Springer.

3. Bauer-Wu, S., Lhundup, T., Tidwell, T., Lhadon, T., Ozawa-de Silva, C., Dolma, J., et al. (2014). Tibetan medicine for cancer. *Integrative Cancer Therapies, 13*(6), 502–512.

4. Chaoul, A., Milbury, K., Spelman, A., Basen-Engquist, K., Hall, M. H., Wei, Q., et al. (2018). Randomized trial of Tibetan yoga in patients with breast cancer undergoing chemotherapy. *Cancer, 124*, 36–45.

5. Adams, V., Schrempf, M., & Craig, S. E. (Ed.). (2013). *Medicine between science and religion: Explorations on Tibetan grounds.* New York: Berghahn Books.

6. Craig, S. R. (2012). *Healing elements: Efficacy and the social ecologies of Tibetan medicine.* Berkeley, CA: University of California Press.

7. Finckh, E. (1980). Tibetan medicine: Theory and practice. In M. Aris & Aung Sang Suu Kyi (Eds.), *Tibetan studies in honor of Hugh Richardson.* Warminster: Aris and Phillips.

8. Kloos, S. (2013). How Tibetan medicine became a "medical system." *East Asian Science, Technology and Society, 7*(3), 381–395.

9. Loizzo, J. J., Blackhall, L. J., & Rapgay, L. (2009). Tibetan medicine: A complementary science of optimal health. *New York Academy of Sciences, 1172*, 218–230.

10. Ozawa De Silva, C., & Ozawa De Silva, B. R. (2011). Mind/body theory and practice in Tibetan medicine and Buddhism. *Body and Society, 17*(1), 95–119.

11. Cameron, M. E., Torkelson, C., Haddow, S., Namdul, T., Prasek, A., & Gross, C. R. (2012). Tibetan medicine and integrative health. *EXPLORE: The Journal of Science and Healing, 8*(3), 158–171.

12. Lindquist, R., Tracy, M. F., & Snyder, M. (2018). *Complementary & alternative therapies in nursing* (8th Ed.). New York: Springer.

13. Baumann, S. L., Murphy, D. C., & Ganzer, C. A. (2015). A study of graduate nursing students' reflections on the art of Tibetan medicine. *Nursing Science Quarterly*, 28(2), 156–161.

14. van Vugt, M. K., Moye, A., Pollock, J., Johnson, B., Bonn-Miller, M. O., Gyatso, K., et al. (2019). Tibetan Buddhist monastic debate: Psychological and neuroscientific analysis of a reasoning-based analytical meditation practice. *Progress in Brain Research, 244*, 233–253.

15. Pintado, S. (2019). Changes in body awareness and self-compassion in clinical psychology trainees through a mindfulness program. *Complementary Therapies in Clinical Practice, 34*, 229–234.

16. Earl E. Bakken Center for Spirituality & Healing, University of Minnesota. (2019). *Learning modules for healthcare professionals.* Retrieved from https://www.csh.umn.edu/education/online-learning-modules-resources/online-learning-modules.

17. Cameron, M. E., & Cheung, C. K. (2018). *Yoga.* In R. Lindquist, M. F. Tracy, & M. Snyder (Eds.). *Complementary/alternative therapies in nursing* (8th Ed.) (chap. 9). New York: Springer.

18. Fernando, A., Rea, C., & Malpas, P. J. (2018). Compassion from a palliative care perspective. *New Zealand Medical Journal, 131*(1468), 25–32.

19. Ferrari, M., Yap, K., Scott, N., Einstein, D. A., & Ciarrochi, J. (2018). Self-compassion moderates the perfectionism and depression link in both adolescence and adulthood. PLoS ONE [Electronic Resource]. 13(2):e0192022.

20. McClelland, L. E., Gabriel, A. S., & DePuccio, M. J. (2018). Compassion practices, nurse well-being, and ambulatory patient experience ratings. *Medical Care, 56*(1), 4–10.

21. Hintsanen, M., Gluschkoff, K., Dobewall, H., Cloninger, C. R., Keltner, D., Saarinen, A., et al. (2019). Parent-child-relationship quality predicts offspring dispositional compassion in adulthood: A prospective follow-up study over three decades. *Developmental Psychology, 55*, 216–225.

22. Monteiro, F., Fonseca, A., Pereira, M., Alves, S., & Canavarro, M. C. (2019). What protects at-risk postpartum women from developing depressive and anxiety symptoms? The role of acceptance-focused processes and self-compassion. *Journal of Affective Disorders, 246*, 522–529.

23. Tirgari, B., Azizzadeh, Forouzi, M., & Ebrahimpour, M. (2019). Relationship between posttraumatic stress disorder and compassion satisfaction, compassion fatigue, and burnout in Iranian psychiatric nurses. *Journal of Psychosocial Nursing & Mental Health Services, 57*, 39–47.

24. Papadopoulos, I., Taylor, G., Ali, S., Aagard, M., Akman, O., Alpers, L. M., et al. (2017). Exploring nurses' meaning and experiences of compassion:

An international online survey involving 15 countries. *Journal of Transcultural Nursing, 28*, 286–295.

25. Straughair, C. (2019). Cultivating compassion in nursing: A grounded theory study to explore the perceptions of individuals who have experienced nursing care as patients. *Nurse Education in Practice, 35*, 98–103.

26. Tierney, S., Seers, K., Tutton, E., & Reeve, J. (2017). Enabling the flow of compassionate care: A grounded theory study. *BMC Health Services Research, 17*, 174.

27. Barron, K., Deery, R., & Sloan, G. (2017). Community mental health nurses and compassion: An interpretative approach. *Journal of Psychiatric & Mental Health Nursing, 24*, 211–220.

28. Kalsang, T. (2016). *Cultivation and conservation of endangered medicinal plants: Tibetan medicinal plants for health*. Dharamsala, India: Men-Tsee-Khang.

29. Norbu, T. (2016). *Encyclopedia of myriad herbs: Medicinal herbs in the Tibetan medical tradition*, vol. 2 (T. Zompa & T. Samdup, Trans.). Dharamsala, India: Men-Tsee-Khang.

30. Namdul, T., Sood, A., Ramakrishnan, L., Pandey, R. M., & Moorthy, D. (2003). Systematic review of herbs and dietary supplements for glycemic control in diabetes. *Diabetes Care, 26*, 1277–1294.

31. Zhao, J. Q., Wang, Y. M., Yang, Y. L., Zeng, Y., Mei, L. J., Shi, Y. P., et al. (2017). Antioxidants and alpha-glucosidase inhibitors from "Liucha" (young leaves and shoots of *Sibiraea laevigata*). *Food Chemistry, 230*, 117–124.

32. Husted, C., & Dhondup, L. (2009). Tibetan medical interpretation of myelin lipids and multiple sclerosis. *Annals of the New York Academy of Science, 1172*, 278–296.

33. Stewart, M., Morling, J. R., & Maxwell, H. (2016). *Padma 28* for intermittent claudication. Cochrane Database of Systematic Reviews, 3, 007371.

34. Feng, C., Wang, W., Ye, J., Li, S., Wu, Q., Yin, D., et al. (2017). Polyphenol profile and antioxidant activity of the fruit and leaf of *vaccinium glaucoalbum* from the Tibetan Himalayas. *Food Chemistry*, 219, 490–495.

35. Chu, B., Chen, C., Li, J., Chen, X., Li, Y., Tang, W., et al. (2017). Effects of Tibetan turnip (*Brassica rapa L.*) on promoting hypoxia-tolerance in healthy humans. *Journal of Ethnopharmacology, 195*, 246–254.

36. Choedon, T., Mathan, G., & Kumar, V. (2015). The traditional Tibetan medicine Yukyung Karne. *BMC Complementary & Alternative Medicine, 15*, 182.

37. Kou, Y., Li, Y., Ma, H., Li, W., Li, R., & Dang, Z. (2016). Uric acid lowering effect of Tibetan medicine *RuPeng 15*. *Journal of Traditional Chinese Medicine, 36*(2), 205–210.

38. Bassa, L. M., Jacobs, C., Gregory, K., Henchey, E., Ser-Dolansky, J., & Schneider, S. S. (2016). *Rhodiola crenulata*. *Phytomedicine, 23*(1), 87–94.

39. Fan, H., Li, T., Gong, N., & Wang, Y. (2016). *Shanzhiside methylester*. Neuropharmacology, *101*, 98–109.

40. Zhou, Y., Li, Z., Tang, F., & Ge, R. (2016). Proteomics annotate therapeutic properties of a traditional Tibetan medicine—Tsantan Sumtang targeting and regulating multiple perturbed pathways. *Journal of Ethnopharmaology*, 181, 108–117.

41. Earl E. Bakken Center for Spirituality & Healing. (2019). *Constitutional Self-Assessment Tool (CSAT) and Lifestyle Guidelines Tool (LGT)*. Retrieved from https://www.csh.umn.edu/education/focus-areas/tibetan-medicine/assessment-and-guidelines-tools.

42. Bonamer, J. R., & Aquino-Russell, C. (2019). Self-care strategies for professional development: Transcendental Meditation reduces compassion fatigue and improves resilience for nurses. *Journal for Nurses in Professional Development, 35*, 93–97.

43. Hanson, M. M. (2018). Rx: Walk in the forest: Shinrin-Yoku's holistic healing effects. *Journal of Alternative and Complementary Medicine, 24*(8), 745–747.

44. Mao, G. X., Cao, Y. B., Yang, Y., Chen, Z. M., Dong, J. H., Chen, S. S., et al. (2018). Additive benefits of twice forest bathing trips in elderly patients with chronic heart failure. *Biomedical & Environmental Sciences, 31(*2), 159–162.

45. Takayama, N., Fujiwara, A., Saito, H., & Horiuchi, M. (2017). Management effectiveness of a secondary coniferous forest for landscape appreciation and psychological restoration. *International Journal of Environmental Research & Public Health [Electronic Resource], 14*.

46. Minnesota Legislature, Office of the Revisor of Statutes. (2018). *2018 Minnesota Statutes, Chapter 146A. Complementary and alternative health care practices*. Retrieved from https://www.revisor.mn.gov/statutes/cite/146A.

47. Sallon, S., Namdul, T., Dolma, S., Dorjee, P., Dolma, D., Sadutshang, T., et al. (2006). Mercury in traditional Tibetan medicine. *Human & Experimental Toxicology, 25*(7), 405–412.

48. Zhou, L. L., Chen, H. J., He, Q. Q., Li, C., Wei, L. X., & Shang, J. (2019). Evaluation of hepatotoxicity potential of a potent traditional Tibetan medicine Zuotai. *Journal of Ethnopharmacology, 234*, 112–118.

49. Sallon, S., Dory, Y., Barghouthy, Y., Tamdin, T., Sangmo, R., Tashi, J., et al. (2017). Is mercury in Tibetan medicine toxic? Clinical, neurocognitive and biochemical results of an initial cross-sectional study. *Experimental Biology & Medicine, 242*, 316–332.

Bibliography

Aristotle. (2012). *Aristotle's Nicomachean Ethics: A new translation* (R. C. Bartlett & S. E. Collins, Trans.). Chicago: University of Chicago Press.

Bradley, T. S. (2013). *Principles of Tibetan medicine: What it is, how it works, and what it can do for you.* Philadelphia: Singing Dragon.

Cameron, M. (1982). *Hello, I'm God and I'm here to help you.* New York: Warner.

Cameron, M. E. (2004). Ethical listening as therapy: Legal and ethical issues. *Journal of Professional Nursing, 20*(3), 141–142.

Cameron, M. E. (2002). *Karma & happiness: A Tibetan odyssey in ethics, spirituality, and healing* (Foreword by His Holiness the Dalai Lama). New York: Rowman & Littlefield.

Cameron, M. E. (1993). *Living with AIDS: Experiencing ethical problems* (Foreword, E. D. Pellegrino). Newbury Park, CA: Sage (based on PhD dissertation).

Cameron, M. E. (2018). *Systems of care; Sowa Rigpa: The Tibetan knowledge of healing.* In R. Lindquist, M. F. Tracy, & M. Snyder (Eds.), *Complementary/ Alternative Therapies in Nursing* (8th Ed.) (pp. 63–77). New York: Springer.

Cameron, M. E., Torkelson, C., Haddow, S., Namdul, T., Prasek, A., & Gross, C. (2012, May/June). Tibetan medicine and integrative health: Validity testing and refinement of the Constitutional Self-Assessment Tool and Lifestyle Guidelines Tool. *EXPLORE: The Journal of Science and Healing, 8*(3), 158–171.

Chenagtsang, N. (2017). *Sowa Rigpa points: Point study in traditional Tibetan medicine.* New York: Sky Press, Tibet House US.

Chenagtsang, N. (2017). *The Tibetan book of health: Sowa Rigpa, the science of healing* (Preface by R. Thurman). New York: Sky Press, Tibet House US.

Coleman, G., & Jinpa, T. (Ed.). (2007). *The Tibetan Book of the Dead: First complete translation* (Foreword by His Holiness the Dalai Lama). New York: Penguin Group.

Dakpa, T. (2007). *Science of healing: A comprehensive commentary on the Root Tantra and diagnostic techniques of Tibetan medicine.* Pittsburgh, PA: Dorrance.

Dalai Lama. (2002). *Advice on dying and living a better life* (J. Hopkins, Trans. & Ed.). New York: Atria Books.

Dalai Lama. (2015). *Beyond religion: Ethics for a whole world.* New York: Harper Element.

Dalai Lama. (2005). *Essence of the Heart Sutra: The Dalai Lama's heart of wisdom teachings* (G. T. Jinpa, Trans.). Boston: Wisdom Publications.

Dalai Lama. (2013). *Kindness, clarity, and insight* (J. Hopkins & E. Napper, Trans. & Eds.). Ithaca, NY: Snow Lion.

Dalai Lama. (2011). *A profound mind: Cultivating wisdom in everyday life* (V. Vreeland, Ed.; Afterword, R. Gere). New York: Harmony.

Dalai Lama. (2005). *The universe in a single atom: How science and spirituality can serve our world.* New York: Morgan Road.

Dalai Lama & Chan, V. (2012). *The wisdom of compassion: Stories of remarkable encounters and timeless insights.* New York: Riverhead.

Dalai Lama & Chan, V. (2004). *The wisdom of forgiveness: Intimate conversations and journeys.* New York: Riverhead.

Dalai Lama & Cutler, H. C. (2009). *The art of happiness.* New York: Riverhead.

Dalai Lama, Tutu, D., & Abrams, D. (2016). *The book of joy: Lasting happiness in a changing world.* London: Hutchinson.

Deane, S. (2018). *Tibetan medicine, Buddhism and psychiatry: Mental health and healing in a Tibetan exile community.* Durham, NC: Carolina Academic Press.

Dhonden, Y. (2000). *Healing from the source: The science and lore of Tibetan medicine.* Ithaca, NY: Snow Lion.

Dhonden, Y. (2000). *Health through balance: An introduction to Tibetan medicine.* Ithaca, NY: Snow Lion.

Dorjee, P., Jones, J., & Moore, T. (2005). *Heal your spirit, heal yourself: The spiritual medicine of Tibet.* London: Watkins.

Drungtso, T. T. (2007). *Basic concepts of Tibetan medicine: A guide to understanding Tibetan medical science.* Dharamsala, India: Drungtso.

Drungtso, T. T. (2006). *Healing power of mantra: The wisdom of Tibetan healing science.* Dharamsala, India: Drungtso.

Evans-Wentz, W. Y. (1960). *The Tibetan Book of the Dead (The after-death experiences on the bardo plane, according to Lama Kazi Dawa-Samdup's English rendering).* New York: Oxford University Press.

Forde, R. Q. (2008). *The book of Tibetan medicine: How to use Tibetan healing for personal wellbeing* (Foreword by H. H. the 17th Karmapa). London: Gaia.

Goleman, D. (2004). *Destructive emotions: How can we overcome them? A scientific dialogue with the Dalai Lama.* New York: Bantam Books.

Gonpo, Y. Y. (1888). *Gyueshi.* Lhasa: Chakpori Press.

Gonpo, Y. Y. (2015a). *Root Trantra and explanatory Tantra (Gyueshi)* (T. Paljor, P. Wangdu, & S. Dolma, Trans.). Dharamsala, India: Men-Tsee-Khang.

Gonpo, Y. Y. (2015b). *Subsequent Tantra (Gyueshi)* (T. Paljor, Trans.). Dharamsala, India: Men-Tsee-Khang.

Gyal, Y. (2006). *Tibetan medical dietary book: Vol. I. Potency & preparation of vegetables* (T. Namdul, Trans. & Ed.). Dharamsala, India: *Men-Tsee-Khang.*

Gyatso, D. S. (2010). *Mirror of beryl* (G. Kilty, Trans.). Boston: Wisdom Publications.

Gyatso, J. (2017). *Being human in a Buddhist world: An intellectual history of medicine in early modern Tibet.* New York: Columbia University Press.

Gyatso, T., & Hakim, C. (2010). *Essentials of Tibetan traditional medicine.* Berkeley, CA: North Atlantic.

Hofer, T. (2018). *Medicine and memory in Tibet: Amchi physicians in the age of reform.* Seattle: University of Washington Press.

Jinpa, T. (2015). *A fearless heart: How the courage to be compassionate can transform our lives.* New York: Avery.

Kabat-Zinn, J., & Davidson, R. J. (Ed.). (2013). *The mind's own physician: A scientific dialogue with the Dalai Lama and the healing power of meditation.* Oakland, CA: New Harbinger.

Khandro, C. (2003). *P'howa Commentary: Instructions for the practice of consciousness transference as revealed by Rigdzin Longsal Nyingpo.* Varanasi, India: Pilgrims Publishing.

Kloos, S. (2013). How Tibetan medicine became a "medical system." *East Asian Science, Technology and Society, 7*(3), 381–395.

Kreitzer, M. J., & Kiothan, M. (2014). *Integrative nursing.* New York: Oxford University Press.

Lindquist, R., Tracy, M. F., & Snyder, M. (2018). *Complementary & alternative therapies in nursing* (8th Ed.). New York: Springer.

Lopez, D. S. (2011). *The Tibetan* Book of the Dead. Princeton, NJ: Princeton University Press.

Mager, S. (2018). *Traditional Tibetan medicine guide: Overview of the most integrated medical system on the planet.* Woodbury, MN: Llewellyn Worldwide.

Men-Tsee-Khang. (2017). *Fundamentals of Tibetan medicine.* Dharamsala, India: Author.

Norbu, T. (2016). *Encyclopedia of myriad herbs: Medicinal herbs in the Tibetan medical tradition* (T. Zompa & T. Samdup, Trans.). Dharamsala, India: *Men-Tsee-Khang.*

Padmasambhava. (2005). *The Tibetan Book of the Dead: First complete translation.* Commentary by HH the Dalai Lama (revealed by T. K. Lingpa; G. Dorje, Ed.; G. Coleman with T. Jinpa, Trans.). New York: Penguin.

Phuntsok, T., & Lhamo, T. (2009). *Study in the elements of Tibetan medicine.* Beijing: China Tibetology Publishing House.

Plato. (1968). *The republic of Plato* (A. Bloom, Trans.). New York: Basic Books.

Ravishankar, S. S. (2016). *Patanjali Yoga sutras.* Bangalore, India: Sri Publications Trust, India.

Rinpoche, C. N., & Shlim, D. R. (2015). *Medicine and compassion: A Tibetan lama and an American doctor on how to provide care with compassion and wisdom.* Somerville, MA: Wisdom Publications.

Rinpoche, D. T. (2002). *The practice of Tibetan meditation: Exercises, visualizations, and mantras for health and well-being.* Rochester, VT: Inner Traditions.

Rinpoche, G., & Lingpa, K. (2003). *The Tibetan Book of the Dead: The great liberation through hearing in the bardo* (F. Fremantle & Chogyam Trungpa, Trans.). Boston: Shambhala.

Rinpoche, S. (2012). *The Tibetan book of living and dying.* New York: HarperCollins.

Rinpoche, Y. M., & Swanson, E. (2007). *The joy of living: Unlocking the secret and science of happiness.* New York: Harmony Books.

Ryan, M. F., & Jamling, D. (2016). *Healing anxiety: A Tibetan medicine guide to healing anxiety, stress and PTSD.* Northampton, MA: Born Perfect.

Samel, G. (2001). *Tibetan medicine.* London: Little, Brown.

Saxer, M. (2013). *Manufacturing Tibetan medicine: The creation of an industry and the moral economy of Tibetanness.* New York: Berghahn Books.

Schachter-Shalomi, Z., & Miller, R. S. (1997). *From age-ing to sage-ing: A profound new vision of growing older.* New York: Warner Books.

Shantideva. (2003). *The way of the Bodhisattva* (Padmakara Translation Group, Trans.). Boston: Shambhala Classics.

Sherab, T., & Jamling, T. T. (2016). *A concise introduction to Tibetan astrology.* Dharamsala, India: *Men-Tsee-Khang.*

Thondup, T. (2006). *Peaceful death, joyful rebirth: A Tibetan Buddhist guidebook.* Boston: Shambhala.

Wallace, B. A., & Hodel, B. (2011). *Stilling the mind: Shamatha teachings from Dudjom Lingpa's Vajra Essence.* Somerville, MA: Wisdom Publications.

Index

location, 203-204; progressive
condition, 201

Earl E. Bakken Center for
Spirituality and Healing,
University of Minnesota, 9;
faculty, 3, 5-6; Tibetan Healing
Initiative, 6; Tibetan medicine
graduate courses, 6; Yoga and
Tibetan Medicine Focus Area, 6
effectiveness, 258-260; gradual
change, 258; precautions, 258-260
elaborate network, 80; channels and
chakras, 67
energy, 18-22, 149; all phenomena,
52-81, 227, 247-249; *joong-wa-
nya*, 18, 35, 52-55, 197, 247-248;
waves in ocean, 103-104. *See also*
air, earth, fire, space, water
ethics, 3-5, 255; ethical and unethical
behavior, 121; ethics research, 3-4;
heals mind, 105-107; integrity,
8, 43, 150; Plato and Aristotle, 4;
proficiency, 189-190; relationship
to happiness, 17-18, 31-33, 247,
260. *See also* happiness/joy. *See also*
health/wellbeing

forgiveness, 32, 107, 152

Gyueshi, 8, 227, 246; basis of book
and Tibetan medicine, 8; basis
of CSAT and LGT, 37-38;
Buddhism, 114; Code of Ethics,
184-190, 193-196; English
translation, 179-180; *Four Tantra*,
181-184'; organization and
components, 180-181. *See also*
Tibetan medical education

happiness/joy, 1-8, 17-36, 152;
meaningful life, 4, 8, 32, 150,

236, 260; meditation, 260 purpose
of life, 1, 98, 247. *See also* ethics.
See also health/wellbeing. *See also*
mind
health/wellbeing, 1-2, 8, 32; body,
81, 129-148, 197-198, 210-212,
247, 256-257; healing, 28-32,
152-153, 210-211, 255; mind,
22-27, 33, 98-128, 254-256;
relationship to ethics and
spirituality, 3-5, 17-18, 22, 28-32.
See also **baekan, loong,** and **tripa.**
See also balance and imbalance.
See also disease. *See also* ethics. *See
also* suffering
His Holiness the 14th Dalai Lama,
5-6; essence of Tibetan medicine,
260; Foreword for *Karma and
Happiness: A Tibetan Odyssey in
Ethics, Spirituality, and Healing,*
5; *Om Mani Padme Hum,*
96; statement about Tibetan
medicine, 9

Islam, 5

Judaism, 5
justice, 32

karma, 3-4, 18-32, 149, 247;
Doctrine of, 118-119; good
karma, 152; karmic seeds, 33

medical anthropology, 2
medicines, 10-11, 236-240;
composites, 236-237; cooling,
warming, or neutral, 238; correct
medicine and administration,
237-238; pacification or
evacuation, 238-239; research,
251-252; Tibetans Precious Pills,
239-240

About the Authors

Miriam E. Cameron, PhD, MS, MA, RN, is lead faculty, Yoga and Tibetan Medicine Focus Area, and graduate faculty, Earl E. Bakken Center for Spirituality and Healing, University of Minnesota. Cameron worked as a staff nurse, nursing supervisor, and nursing instructor before going to graduate school. Since 1994, she has studied, conducted research, and taught graduate courses about Tibetan medicine, yoga, nursing, and ethics. She has published over 65 journal articles, nine book chapters, three monographs, three internet modules, and three other books including *Karma & Happiness: A Tibetan Odyssey in Ethics, Spirituality, & Healing*, with the foreword by His Holiness the 14th Dalai Lama.

Tenzin Namdul, PhD, DTM, medical anthropologist and experienced Tibetan medicine practitioner, is teaching faculty at the Earl E. Bakken Center for Spirituality and Healing, University of Minnesota. Namdul has conducted Tibetan medicine consultations around the world. He has published research articles and an internet module about Tibetan Medicine, and he translated from Tibetan to English the *Tibetan Medical Dietary Book: Vol. I, Potency & Preparation of Vegetables* by Yangbum Gyal. Previously, he served as faculty and director of research at the Men-Tsee-Khang, the Tibetan Medical Instutite in Dharamsala, India.